Self-assessment picture tests
Medicine
Volume 1

Pierre-Marc Bouloux
BSc MD FRCP

Reader in Endocrinology
Department of Endocrinology
Royal Free Hospital
London

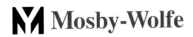 **Mosby-Wolfe**

London • Baltimore • Barcelona • Bogotá • Boston
Buenos Aires • Carlsbad, CA • Chicago • Madrid
Mexico City • Milan • Naples, FL • New York
Philadelphia • St. Louis • Seoul • Singapore
Sydney • Taipei • Tokyo • Toronto • Wiesbaden

Publisher:	**Richard Furn**
Development Editor:	**Jennifer Prast**
Project Manager:	**Linda Horrell, Jane Tozer**
Production:	**Gudrun Hughes**
Index:	**Angela Cottingham**
Layout:	**Lindy van den Berghe**
Cover Design:	**Greg Smith**

ISBN 0 7234 2464 0   Set ISBN 0 7234 2468 3

For full details of all Times Mirror International Publishers Limited titles, please write to Times Mirror International Publishers Limited, Lynton House, 7–12 Tavistock Square, London WC1H 9LB, England.

A CIP catalogue record for this book is available from the British Library.

Preface

Much of clinical practice consists of pattern recognition, and the ability to detect swiftly and interpret physical signs correctly is at the heart of the diagnostic process (and indeed a prequisite for passing clinical examinations!). In these four volumes, I have compiled 800 examples of common and not so common clinical problems covering wide areas of medicine. The format is simple, unambiguous and unpretentious: a photographic plate with a short question, or questions, relating to the physical sign or underlying diagnosis. The aim is to challenge the reader's diagnostic skills. I have annotated the answer in many cases to give the reader some background information about the condition illustrated. These volumes should be seen as an adjunct to existing illustrated textbooks of clinical medicine such as Forbes/Jackson *Color Atlas and Text of Clinical Medicine,* 2nd edition.

Acknowledgements

I would like to acknowledge the wonderful assistance given to me by the Department of Medical Illustrations at the Royal Free Hospital School of Medicine, and the excellent support of Miss Patsy Coskeran in assembling the material.

To Jane, Dominic, Matthew, Natalie and my late brother Alain

1 ▶

This man presented to his general practitioner complaining of cramps.

(a) What is the most likely diagnosis?

(b) List two essential investigations.

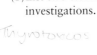

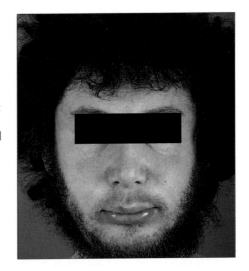

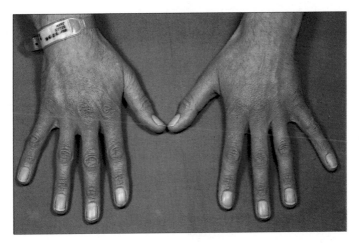

▲ 2

These are the hands of a patient who was under investigation by an ophthalmologist for monocular diplopia.

(a) What abnormality is shown?

(b) What ocular abnormality may be associated?

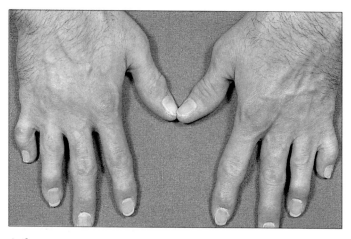

▲ 3
These are the hands of the patient under investigation for a persistently low serum calcium.
(a) What is the likely underlying diagnosis?
(b) What is the molecular explanation for this condition?

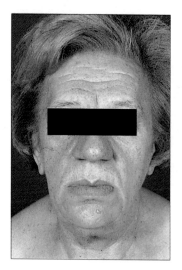

◄ 4
This patient presented with sleep apnoea and snoring.
(a) What is the diagnosis?
(b) List two typical biochemical abnormalities.

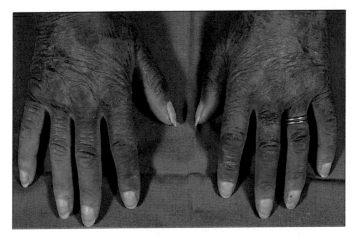

▲ 5

These are the hands of a patient complaining of soreness and increased pigmentation.
(a) What is the diagnosis?
(b) What is the biochemical basis for the condition?

6 ▶

This is the chest of a patient who is under investigation for hypertension.
(a) What is the likely underlying diagnosis?
(b) List four neurological complications of this disease.

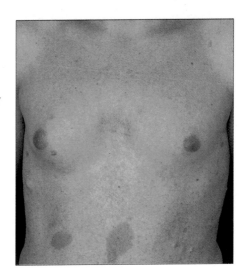

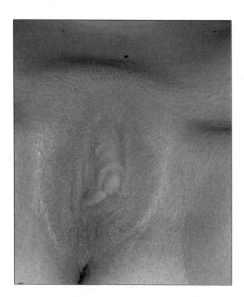

◀ 7
(a) What physical sign is shown?
(b) List two additional physical signs that might be found in this patient?

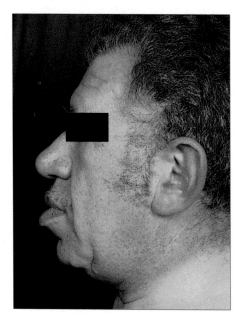

◀ 8
This is the profile of a man who complained of headaches.
(a) What is the diagnosis?
(b) List three cardiovascular complications of this disease.

9 ▶
This lady
complained of itchy
irritating nodules
on the anterior
aspects of her legs.
A scar in the base of
the neck was noted.
(a) What lesion is
    shown?
(b) How is it
    treated?

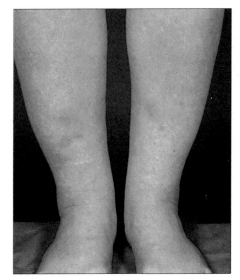

10 ▶
(a) What physical
    sign is shown?
(b) With what
    neurological
    complication
    may it be
    associated?

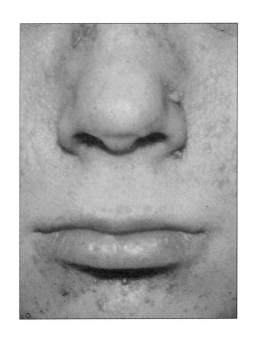

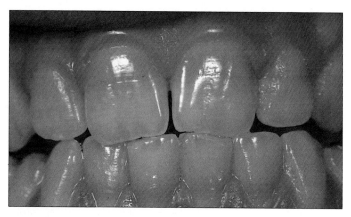

▲ 11

These are the teeth of a child who had been exposed to an antibiotic.

(a) What was the likely antibiotic used?
(b) What is the mechanism of this effect?

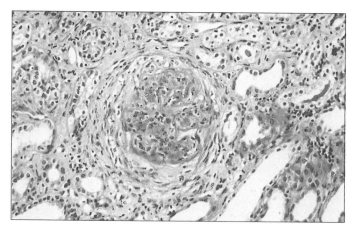

▲ 12

This is a haematoxylin and eosin stain of a renal biopsy from a patient with a rapidly progressive renal lesion. What is the diagnosis?

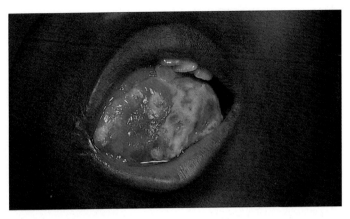

▲ 13

This lesion had been present over a number of months and had been fairly rapidly progressive. What is the likely diagnosis?

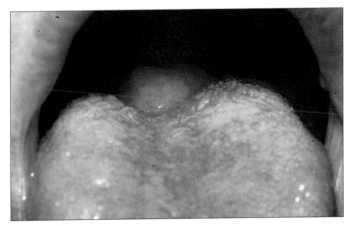

▲ 14

This lump had been present throughout the patient's life.

(a) What is it likely to be?

(b) Suggest a confirmatory investigation.

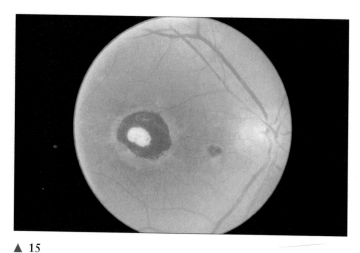

▲ 15
(a) What is the diagnosis?
(b) With what physical sign would it be associated?

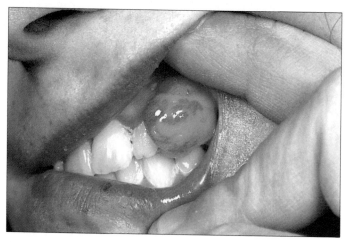

▲ 16
(a) What is this lesion?
(b) What is its treatment?

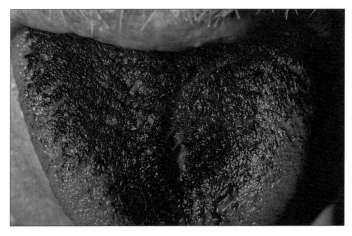

▲ 17
(a) What physical sign is shown?
(b) List two causes.

18 ▶
With what conditions may this discoloration be associated?

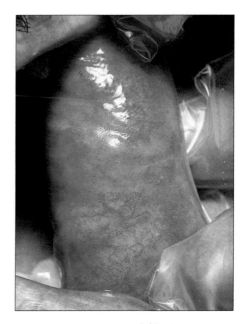

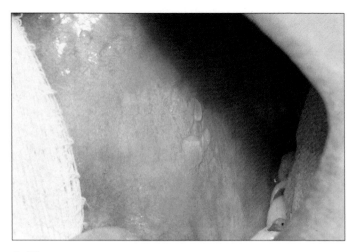

▲ 19
This lesion was associated with other itchy skin lesions. What is the diagnosis?

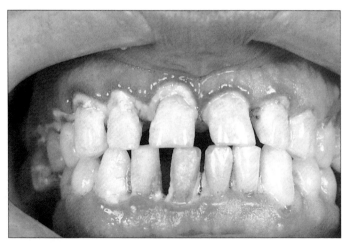

▲ 20
This man was under investigation for chronic anaemia. What physical sign is shown?

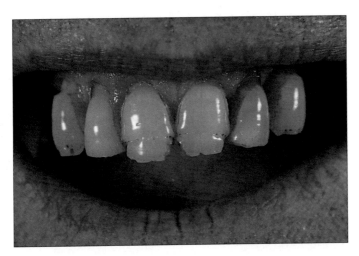

▲ 21
What physical sign is shown, and with what disease is it associated?

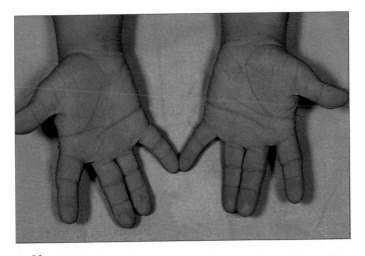

▲ 22
(a) What physical sign is shown?
(b) Cite one confirmatory test.

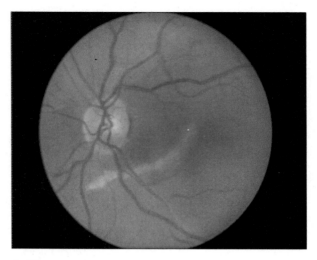

▲ 23
(a) What physical sign is shown?
(b) With what ocular condition may it be associated?

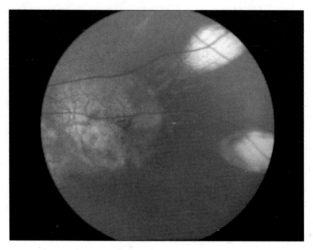

▲ 24
What physical sign is shown?

25 ▶

This is the appearance of the leg of a patient who has bleeding gums.
(a) What is the most likely diagnosis?
(b) List three other complications of the condition.

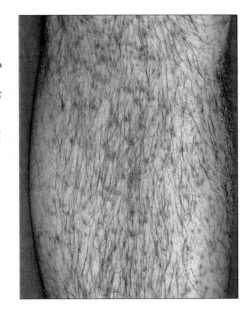

26 ▶

(a) What abnormality is shown?
(b) Are any systemic manifestations expected?

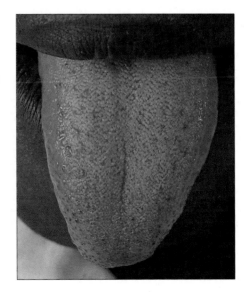

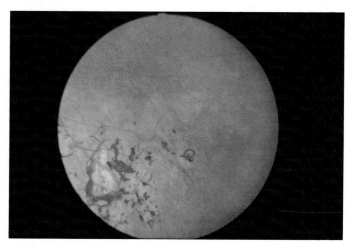

▲ 27
(a) What abnormality is shown?
(b) With what symptoms may the patient present?

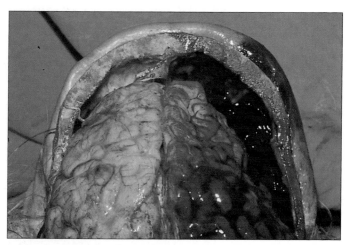

▲ 28
What was the cause of death?

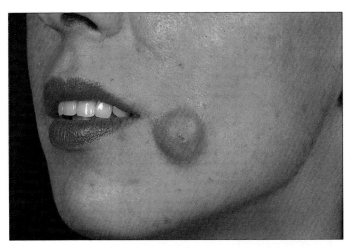

▲ 29
This is the face of a patient who had several such lesions over her body, in addition to osteomas. What diagnosis should be suspected?

30 ▶
What lesion is shown?

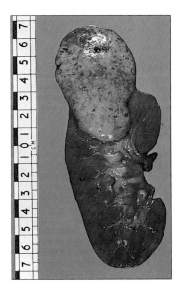

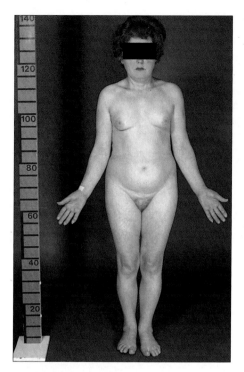

◀ 31
This patient presented with primary amenorrhoea. What is the most likely diagnosis?

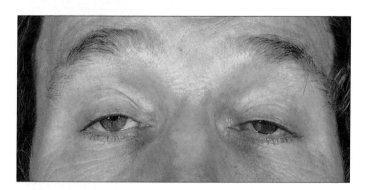

▲ 32
(a) What physical sign is shown?
(b) List three associated conditions.

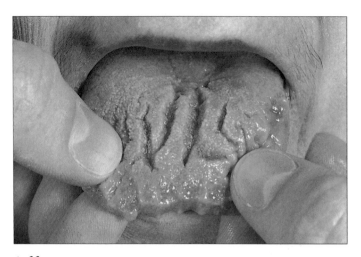

▲ 33
(a) What physical sign is shown?
(b) What treatment is needed?

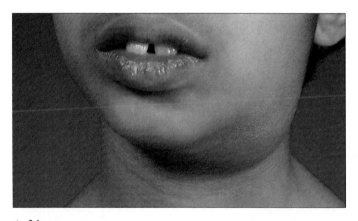

▲ 34
This patient presented with an insidious onset of ill-health and night sweats. There had been loss of weight and the lesion in the angle of the mandible had gradually increased in size over three months and was not tender. There was no lymphadenopathy. What diagnosis should be strongly suspected?

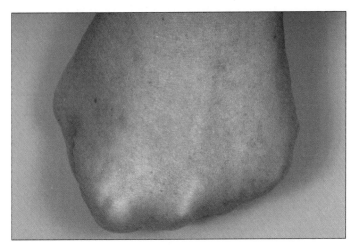

▲ 35
This is the hand of a patient with anosmia. What diagnosis is suggested?

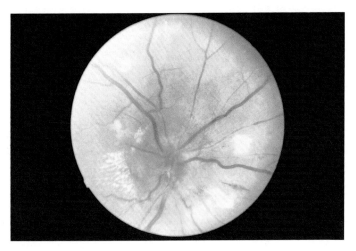

▲ 36
What diagnosis should be strongly suspected with this fundal appearance?

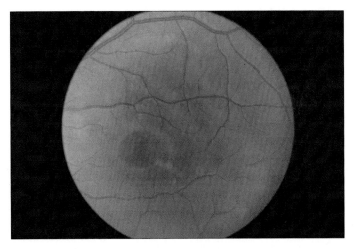

▲ 37
(a) What physical sign is shown?
(b) What is the likely symptom at presentation?

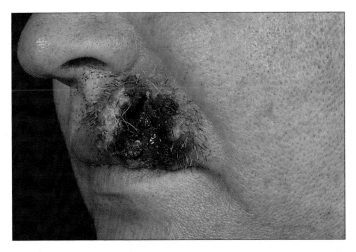

▲ 38
(a) What is the likely cause of this lesion?
(b) List two predisposing factors.

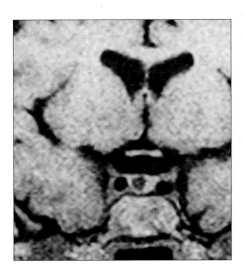

This investigation was carried out in a 27-year-old woman with secondary amenorrhoea and breast discharge.

(a) What investigation is shown?
(b) What abnormality is demonstrated?
(c) What associated biochemical abnormality may be found?
(d) What treatment is indicated?

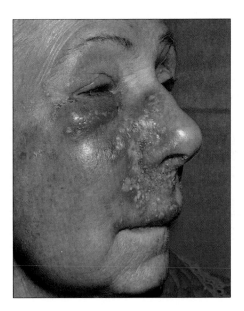

◀ 40
(a) What lesion is shown?
(b) What is the aetiological agent?

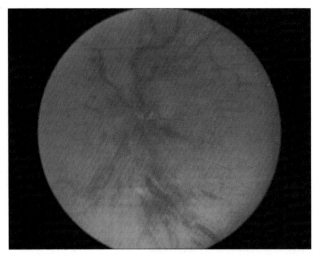

▲ 41
(a) What is the cause of this fundal appearance?
(b) Cite one complication.

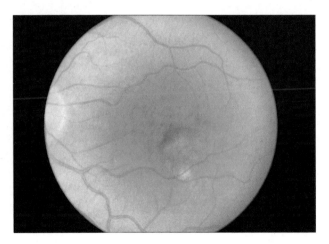

▲ 42
At a routine examination this patient was found to have a scotoma. The lesion in the macula had been expanding in size. What is the most likely diagnosis?

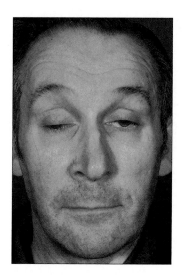

◀ 43
This is the appearance of a man who presented with nasal regurgitation of food and diplopia.
(a) What is the most likely diagnosis?
(b) What outpatient investigation may be performed to diagnose it?

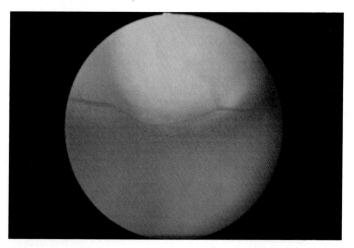

▲ 44
This is the fundal appearance of a patient who complained of rapid onset of loss of vision.
(a) What is the diagnosis?
(b) What specific visual field defect may be present?

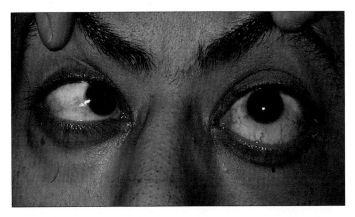

▲ 45

This patient had a nasopharyngeal carcinoma. What physical sign is shown?

46 ▶

These are the legs of a patient who had a normal nutrition and was not known to suffer from any malabsorptive state. There was a family history of the condition, which occurred only in males. What is the diagnosis?

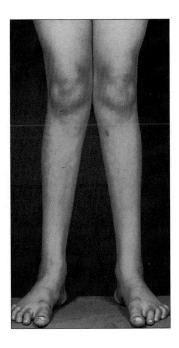

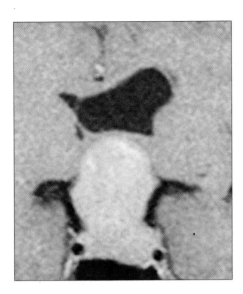

◄ 47
(a) What abnormality is shown?
(b) List two symptoms this patient is likely to have.

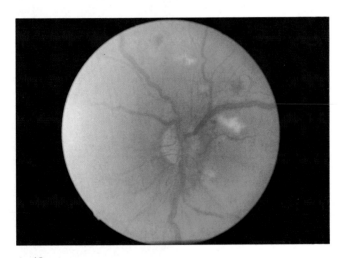

▲ 48
(a) What is the most likely cause of this retinal appearance?
(b) Cite one confirmatory test.

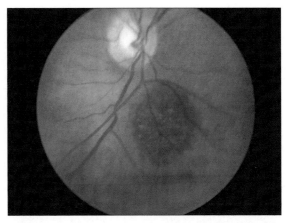

▲ 49

This lesion was picked up on routine fundoscopy. The patient was asymptomatic and had no physical signs.
(a) What is the likely diagnosis?
(b) What action is needed?

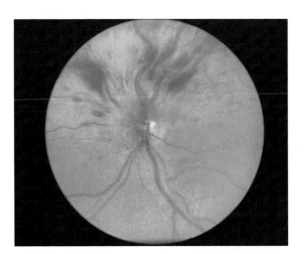

▲ 50

(a) What diagnosis is suggested by this appearance?
(b) List three predisposing causes.

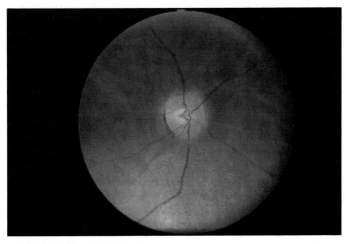

▲ 51

This is the fundal appearance of a patient receiving antimalarial drugs for severe rheumatoid arthritis. The patient presented with blurred vision. What diagnosis is suggested by this appearance?

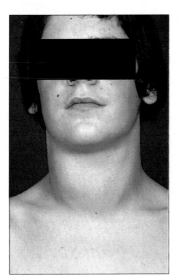

◄ 52

This is the appearance of a young man with a diffuse goitre and sensorineural deafness.

(a) What diagnosis is suggested by these physical signs?

(b) What is the mode of inheritance?

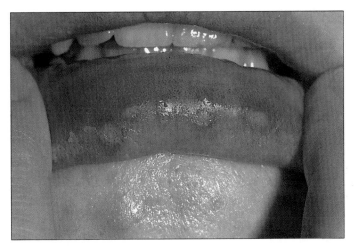

▲ 53

This painful lesion occurred over a matter of days.
(a) What is the most likely diagnosis?
(b) Cite one systemic complications of this condition.

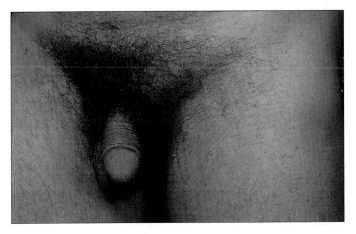

▲ 54

(a) What physical sign is shown?
(b) List two potential complications.

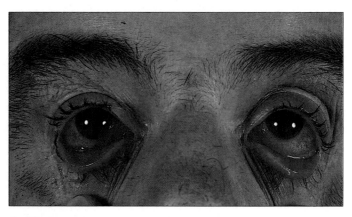

▲ 55
Following a diarrhoeal illness this patient developed a penile discharge and sore eyes. What is the likely diagnosis?

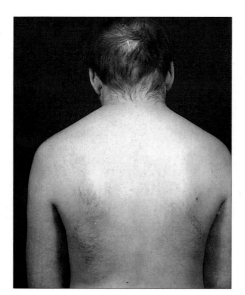

◀ 56
This patient suffered from the phenomenon of hereditary bimanual synkinesis. What diagnosis is suggested by this appearance?

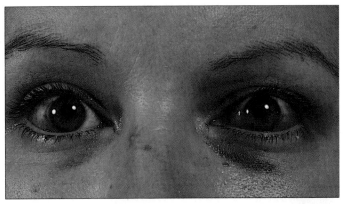

▲ 57

Following a windsurfing holiday, this patient presented with a fever, an intense headache, and a rapid onset of jaundice with conjunctival haemorrhages. Gingival bleeding ensued.
(a) What is the most likely diagnosis?
(b) What is the treatment?

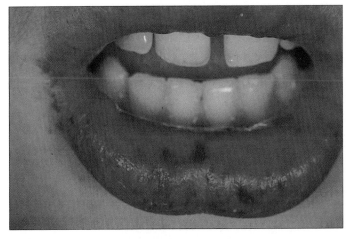

▲ 58

This patient suffered from iron deficiency anaemia. What diagnosis is suggested by this physical sign?

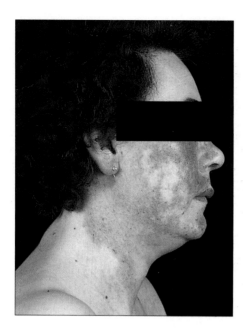

◀ 59
This is the appearance of a patient who underwent resection for a hypernephroma. What diagnosis is suggested by this physical sign?

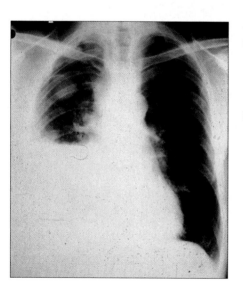

◀ 60
(a) What two radiographic abnormalities are seen on this chest radiograph?
(b) What is the most probable underlying diagnosis?

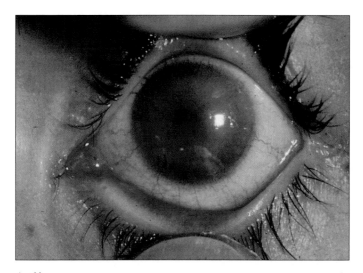

▲ 61
(a) What physical sign is shown?
(b) With what group of diseases is it associated?

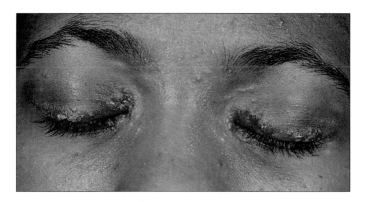

▲ 62
These are the eyes of a patient who complained of a dry
unproductive cough, polyuria, and polydipsia.
(a) What is the likely underlying diagnosis?
(b) List two biochemical abnormalities associated with this condition.

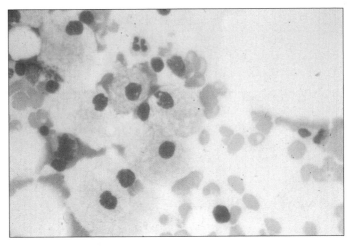

▲ **63**

This is the appearance of the bone marrow of a patient with avascular necrosis of the femoral neck.

(a) What is the diagnosis?

(b) What is the underlying biochemical abnormality?

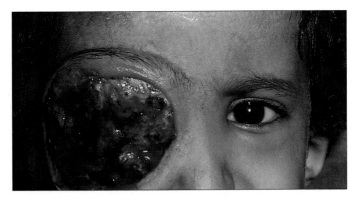

▲ **64**

This is the appearance of a young boy who was losing his vision in both eyes. A sibling had the same condition.

(a) What is the likely diagnosis?

(b) What is the mechanism of disease?

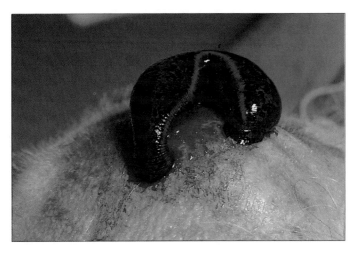

▲ 65
What mode of therapy is demonstrated here?

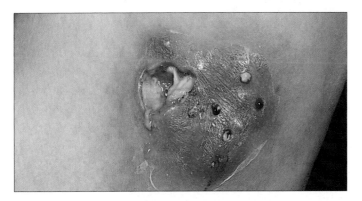

▲ 66
(a) What lesion is shown?
(b) What is the likely organism?

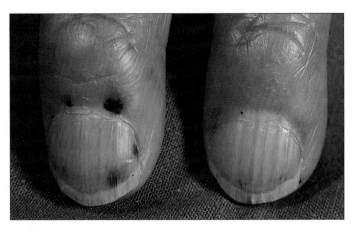

▲ 67
What underlying process is likely to be responsible for these lesions?

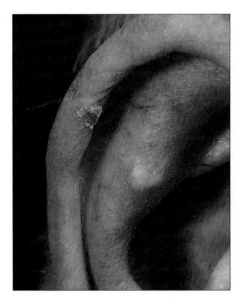

◀ 68
(a) What lesion is shown?
(b) What is the underlying biochemical abnormality?

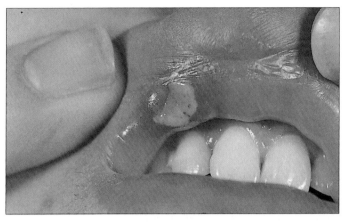

▲ 69

This is one of several lesions which were extremely painful and lasted 7–10 days. They healed completely, but tended to recur in other sites. What is the likely diagnosis?

70 ▶
(a) What physical sign is shown?
(b) List three possible causes.

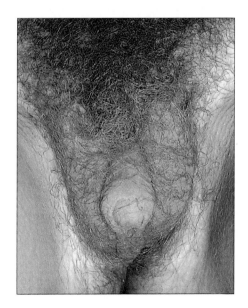

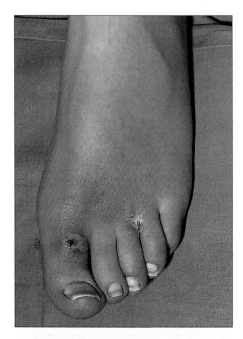

◀ 71
This is the foot of a patient who worked in a shipyard. A few days after this photograph was taken, a central eschar appeared. What is the likely underlying diagnosis?

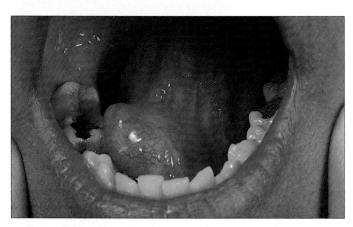

▲ 72
What lesion is shown?

73 ▶
(a) What is the likely
diagnosis?
(b) What HLA
association does
this disease have?

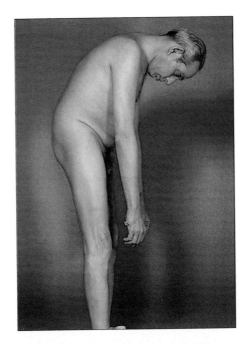

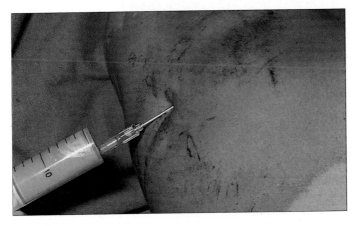

▲ **74**
This needle is aspirating a lymph node. What is the likely
diagnosis?

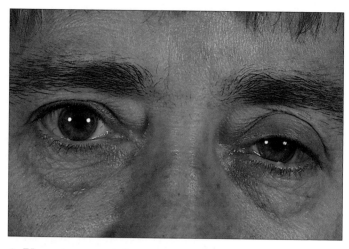

▲ 75
(a) What physical sign is shown?
(b) What are the component parts of this condition?

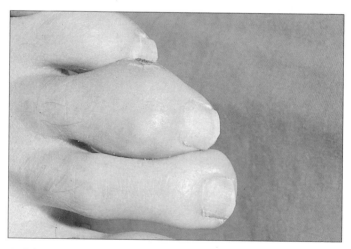

▲ 76
What diagnosis is suggested by this appearance?

77 ▶

This man presented to an endocrine outpatient department with a complaint of primary infertility. The testes were found to be less than 3 ml and firm.

(a) What is the likely underlying diagnosis?

(b) Cite one confirmatory test.

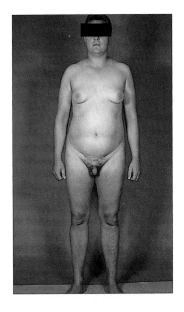

78 ▶

This patient was being treated for a chronic inflammatory condition.

(a) What physical sign is shown?

(b) What therapy is she probably receiving?

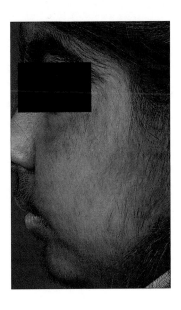

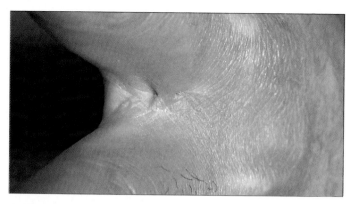

▲ 79

This is the web between the fingers of this man who worked as a hairdresser. What is the likely diagnosis?

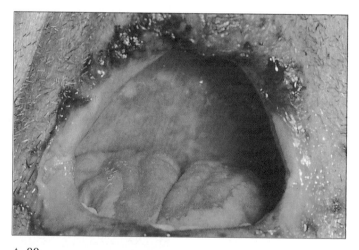

▲ 80

After taking co-trimoxazole this man developed widespread soreness of his lips and mucous membranes.

(a) What is the likely diagnosis?

(b) List three additional causes.

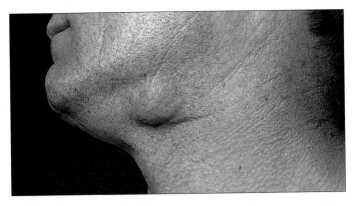

▲ 81
(a) What is the likely cause of this appearance? It has been present for nine weeks.
(b) What investigation is required?

82 ▶
This is the face of a patient complaining of recurrent flushing episodes. There had been some diarrhoea.
(a) What diagnosis is suggested by this appearance?
(b) How should the diagnosis be confirmed?

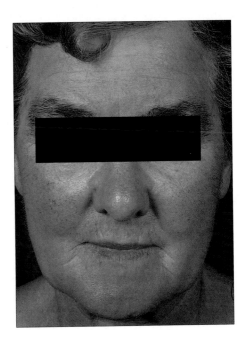

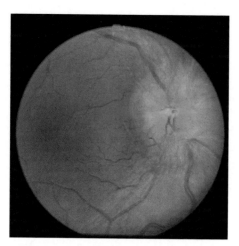

◀ 83
(a) What physical sign is shown?
(b) List three possible causes.

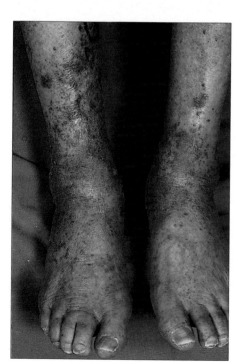

◀ 84
These are the appearance of the legs of a patient who presented with fever and haematuria.
(a) What underlying diagnosis should be considered?
(b) How can the diagnosis be confirmed?

85 ▶

This man complained of diplopia and difficulty swallowing.

(a) What is the likely underlying diagnosis?

(b) What chest complication should be sought?

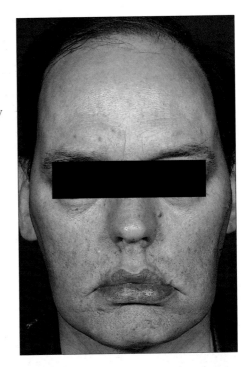

86 ▶

This patient presented with rapid altitudinal field loss. What is the likely diagnosis?

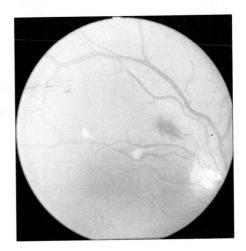

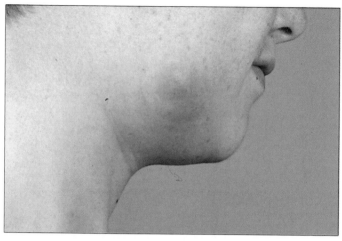

▲ 87
This patient was under investigation for erythema nodosum associated with cervical lymphadenopathy and had otherwise been in good health. He kept several pets at home. Suggest a possible cause for this lymphadenopathy.

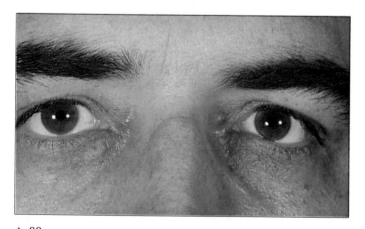

▲ 88
(a) What physical sign is shown?
(b) List two associated diseases.

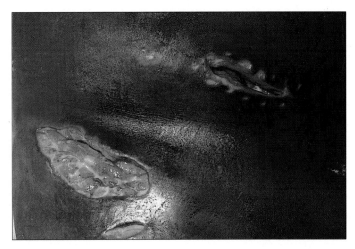

▲ 89
Following an appendicectomy, the wound dehisced and there was a chronic suppurative discharge from a sinus. What diagnosis is suggested?

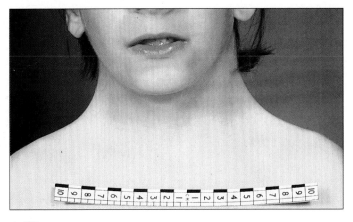

▲ 90
(a) What physical sign is shown?
(b) Cite one diagnostic test.

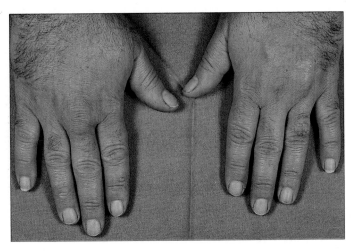

▲ 91

These are the hands of a patient with a family history of premature coronary artherosclerosis. What is the likely diagnosis?

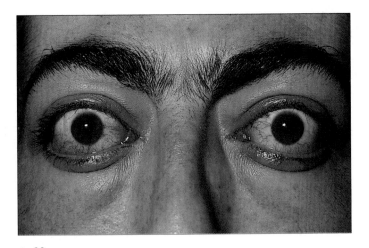

▲ 92

(a) What is the likely diagnosis?
(b) List three additional ocular complications of this condition.

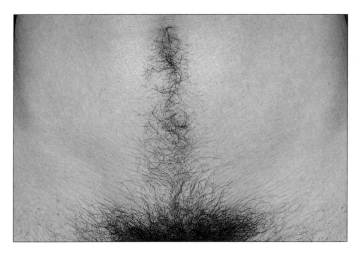

▲ 93

(a) What physical sign is shown? The patient was under investigation for primary infertility.

(b) What is the commonest cause of this abnormality?

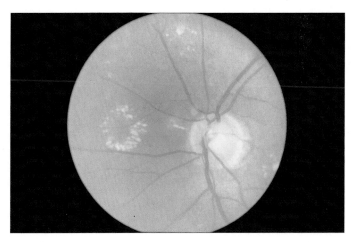

▲ 94

(a) What is the most likely cause of this appearance?

(b) What additional investigations would be required?

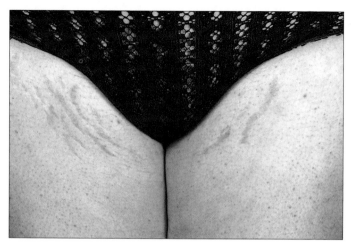

▲ 95
(a) What physical sign is shown?
(b) List two classical biochemical abnormalities.

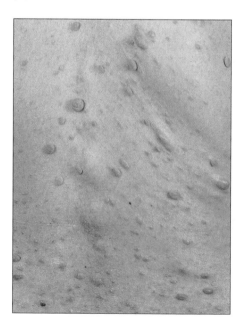

◄ 96
This is the skin of a patient complaining of deafness and ataxia.
(a) What is the likeliest diagnosis?
(b) What is the probable cause of the neurology?

97 ▶
What haematological disorder is suggested by this skull appearance?

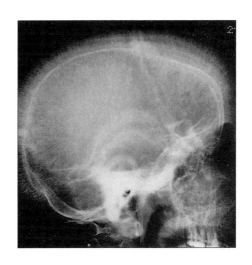

98 ▶
This is the ear of a man complaining of pains in his large joints. What diagnosis is suggested?

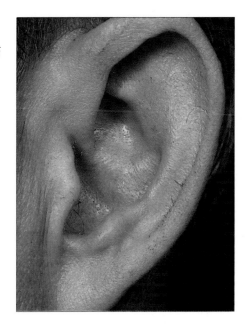

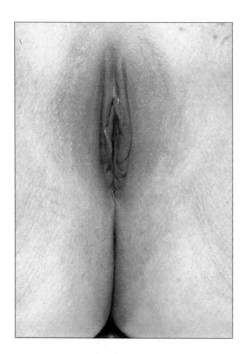

◀ 99
This patient was about to undergo exploration of her inguinal regions for what were thought to be hernias. Although she had full breasts, at no stage had any secondary sexual hair appeared, and she had never menstruated.

(a) What is the most likely underlying diagnosis?
(b) What is the biochemical basis of this condition?

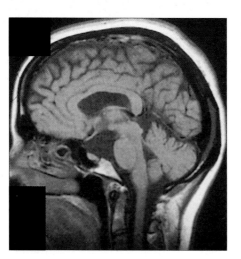

◀ 100
What abnormality is demonstrated in this patient who presented with headaches and disturbed thermoregulation?

▲ 101

This followed a febrile illness associated with considerable leucocytosis. What is the diagnosis?

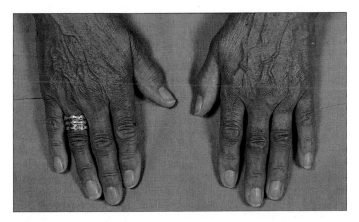

▲ 102

This patient underwent a bilateral adrenalectomy for Cushing's disease 30 years previously. She then noticed that her hands were getting progressively darker. What is the probable underlying cause?

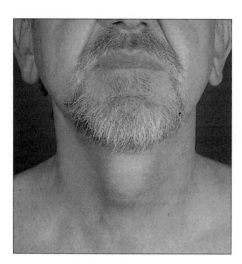

◄ 103
This man complained of a lump in his neck, which had been present ever since he could remember. What is the most likely cause?

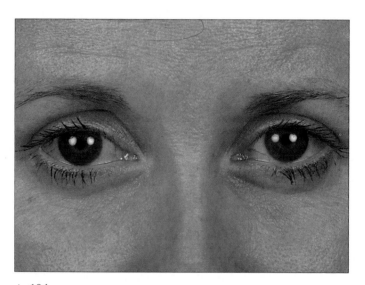

▲ 104
(a) What physical sign is shown?
(b) With what disease is it associated?

105 ▶
What echocardiographic abnormality is shown?

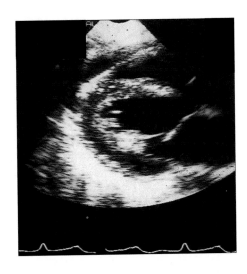

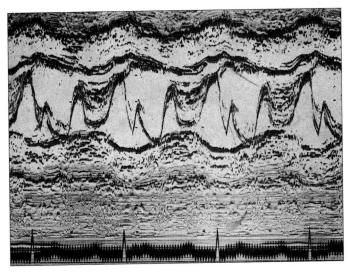

▲ 106
What echocardiographic abnormality is suggested by this appearance?

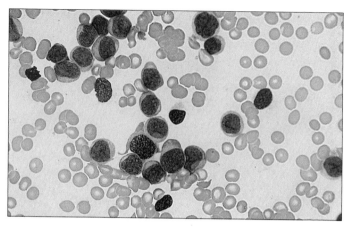

▲ 107

This is the blood film of a patient who presented with anaemia and easy bruising. What is the likely diagnosis?

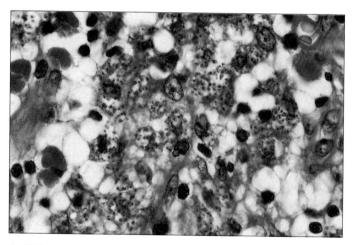

▲ 108

This is the bone marrow smear from a patient suffering from nocturnal fevers, diarrhoea, and lymphadenopathy. The blood film showed pancytopenia. What is the diagnosis?

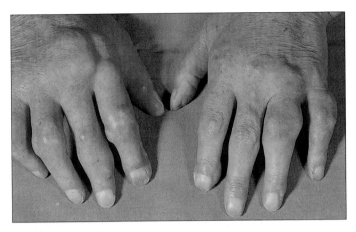

▲ 109
(a) What diagnosis is suggested by these appearances?
(b) What renal complication may supervene?

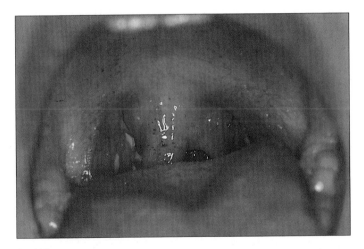

▲ 110
This patient was under investigation for a febrile illness of unknown aetiology associated with severe headaches. What is the most likely diagnosis?

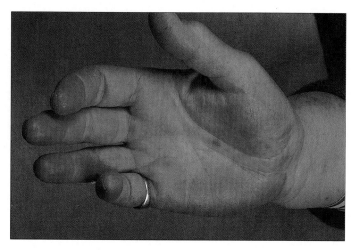

▲ 111
(a) What physical sign is shown?
(b) List three associations.

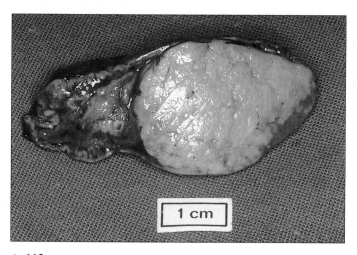

▲ 112
This is an adrenal resection specimen from a patient with moderate hypertension associated with hypokalaemia. What is the diagnosis?

113 ▶
What is the
ophthalmological
diagnosis?

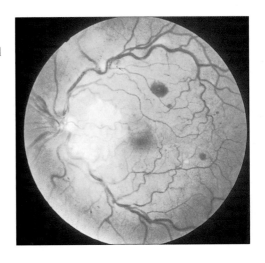

114 ▶
This lesion was
picked up
incidentally in
the eye of a
patient known to
suffer from
chronic epilepsy.
What is the
diagnosis?

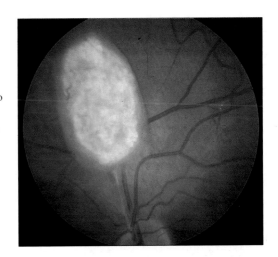

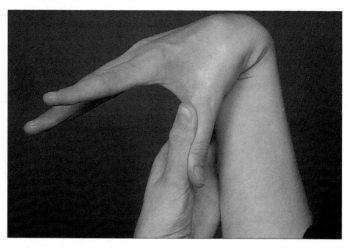

▲ 115
(a) What physical sign is demonstrated?
(b) List two associations.

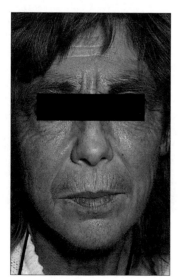

◀ 116
This patient is known to have chronic liver disease and developed hirsutism and darkening of the skin over a one-year period. What diagnosis is suggested?

117 ▶
These are the lesions found on
the skin of an insulin-dependent
diabetic. What is the diagnosis?

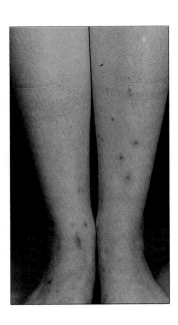

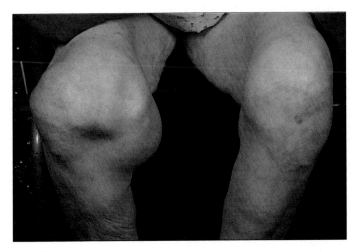

▲ 118
What is the cause of these painless deformities?

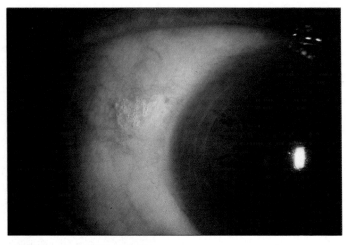

▲ 119
(a) What physical sign is shown?
(b) What is the underlying diagnosis?

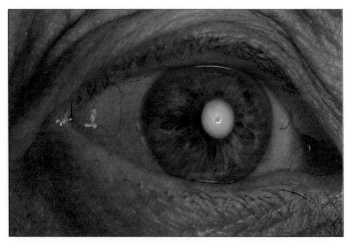

▲ 120
What biochemical abnormality is suggested by this appearance?
(NB There is a flash gun artefact in the pupil.)

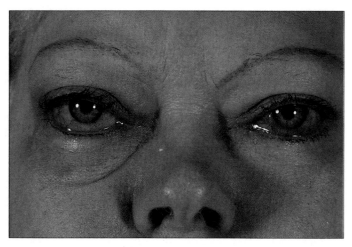

▲ 121
This patient was complaining of pain and grittiness of the eyes.
There had been recent significant weight loss.
(a) What is the most likely diagnosis?
(b) What physical signs are shown?

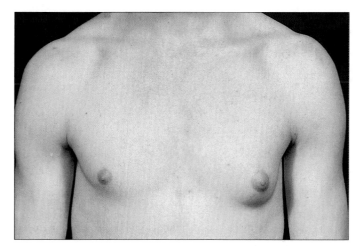

▲ 122
What specific causes should be sought for this physical sign?

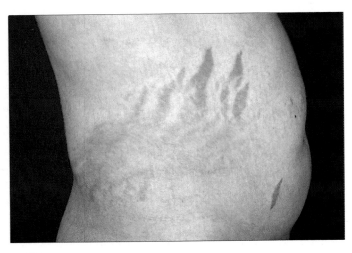

▲ 123
(a) What physical sign is shown?
(b) The patient had mild hyperglycaemia and was hypertensive.
     What is the most likely diagnosis?

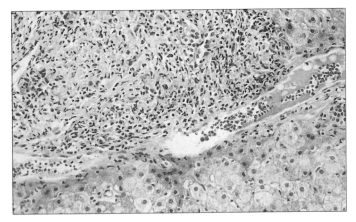

▲ 124
This liver biopsy is taken from a patient with jaundice and intense
pruritus. Her alkaline phosphatase had been known to be elevated
for a six-year period before presentation. What is the diagnosis?

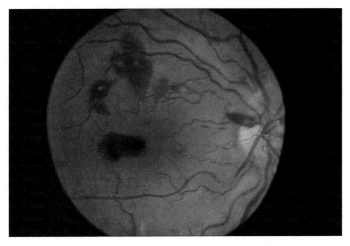

▲ 125

This is the fundal appearance of a patient complaining of weight loss, fever, and haematuria. What is the diagnosis?

126 ▶

These are the legs of a patient who had previously received iodine-131 therapy for thyrotoxicosis. What lesion is shown?

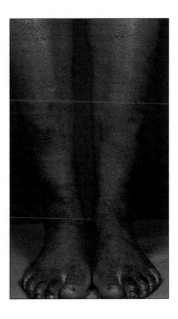

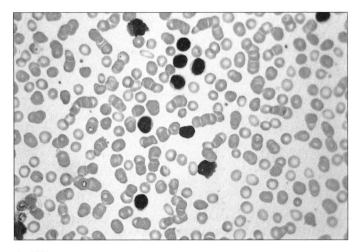

▲ 127

This is a film taken from a patient suffering from lethargy. What is the diagnosis?

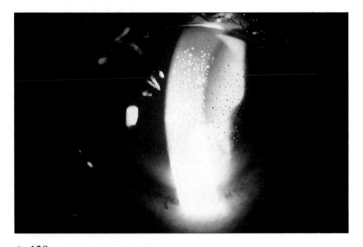

▲ 128

(a) What abnormality is shown on this slit lamp examination?
(b) What investigations are indicated.

129 ▶

These are the legs of a patient with extreme short stature, and severe hypophosphataemia. What is the likely underlying diagnosis?

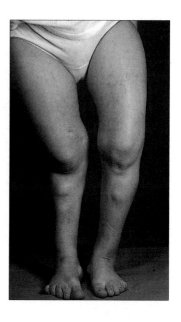

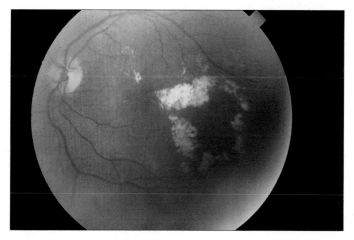

▲ **130**

(a) What abnormality is shown on fundoscopy?
(b) What is the probable underlying diagnosis?

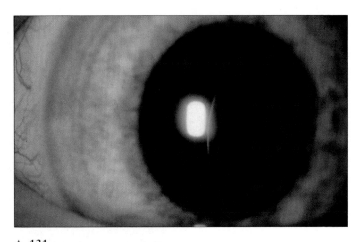

▲ 131
(a) What physical sign is shown?
(b) With what symptom is it characteristically associated?

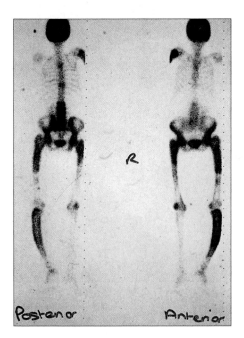

◀ 132
(a) What disease is likely to cause this technetium methylene diphosphonate (MDP) scan appearance?
(b) With what characteristic biochemical abnormality is it associated?

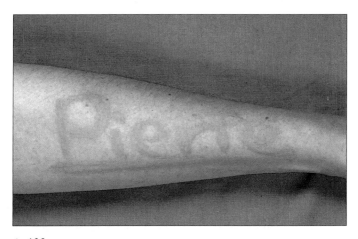

▲ 133
(a) What physical sign is shown?
(b) With what symptoms do patients usually present?

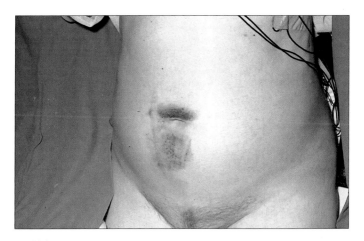

▲ 134
This patient developed sudden severe anaemia on the ward. There was no evidence of blood loss from the upper or lower gastrointestinal tract nor, indeed, from the renal tract. This physical sign appeared after three days. What is the likely cause?

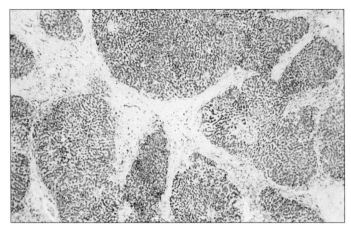

▲ 135

This is a liver biopsy.

(a) What stain has been used?

(b) What is the likely underlying diagnosis?

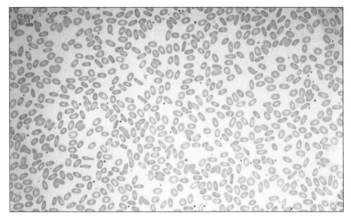

▲ 136

What morphological abnormality of red cells is shown in this film?

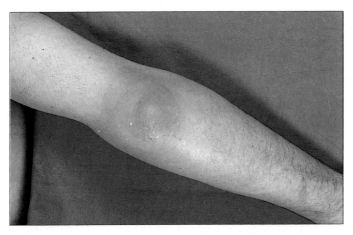

▲ 137
One month after starting treatment for hypertension, this patient developed a painful elbow. What is the likely diagnosis?

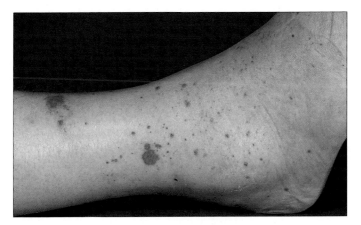

▲ 138
This is the leg of a patient who presented with an asymptomatic rash, but who on routine urine testing was found to have microscopic haematuria. What is the underlying diagnosis?

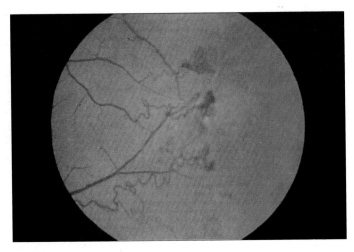

▲ 139
With what haematological condition is this appearance associated?

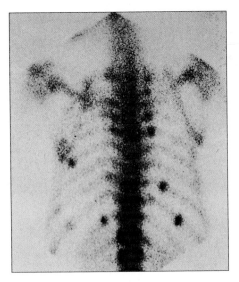

◄ 140
What is the most likely cause of this appearance?

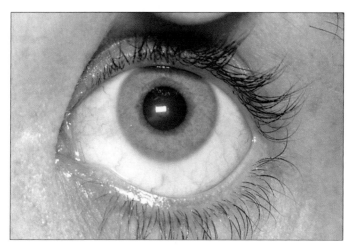

▲ 141

This patient was under investigation for a pancytopenia, and multiple osteopenic fractures of the vertebrae.

(a) What physical sign is shown?

(b) With what disease is it associated?

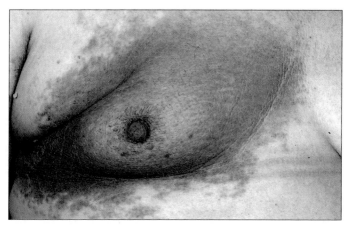

▲ 142

(a) What physical sign is shown?

(b) What are three associated conditions?

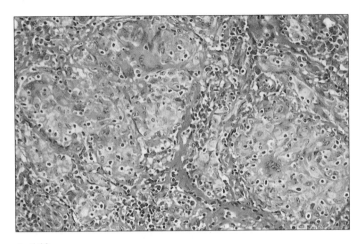

▲ 143
This is the histological appearance of a lymph node removed from a patient with hypocalcaemia.
(a) What abnormality is shown?
(b) What is the likely underlying diagnosis?

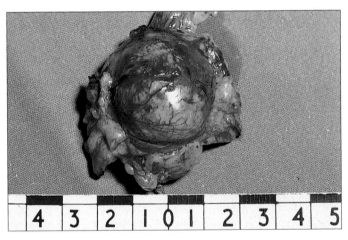

▲ 144
This tumour was removed from a patient with hypertension. What is the likely diagnosis?

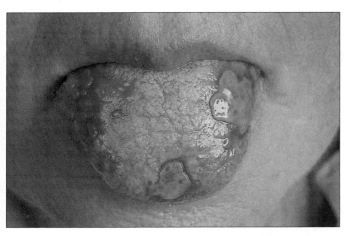

▲ 145
This is the appearance of the tongue of a 45-year-old woman with bloody diarrhoea. She also had arthralgia and a necrotic-looking lesion on the front of her shins. What is the most likely diagnosis?

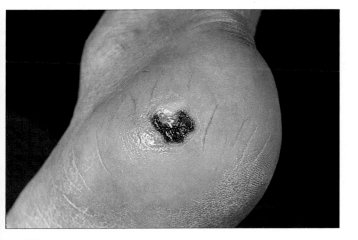

▲ 146
This painless lesion had been present for over two months. What is the most likely underlying diagnosis?

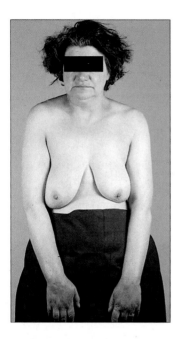

◀ 147
This is a patient who presented with a history of recurrent falls. What diagnosis is suggested by her appearance?

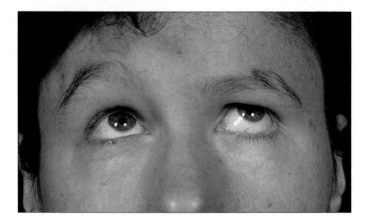

▲ 148
(a) What physical sign is shown?
(b) What are the three possible causes?

149 ▶
List two potential
causes of this
physical sign?

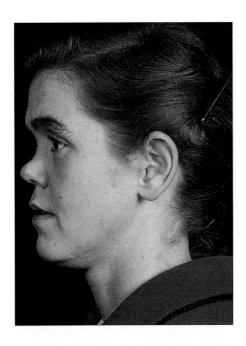

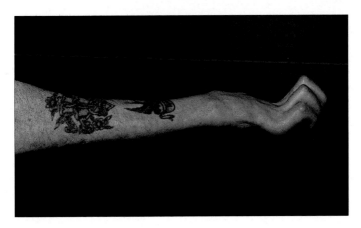

▲ **150**
(a) What lesion is shown?
(b) List two possible causes.

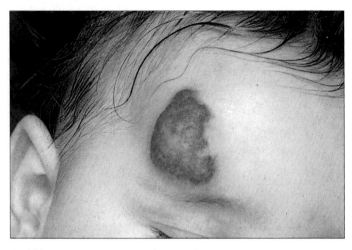

▲ 151
(a) What lesion is shown?
(b) What treatment is appropriate?

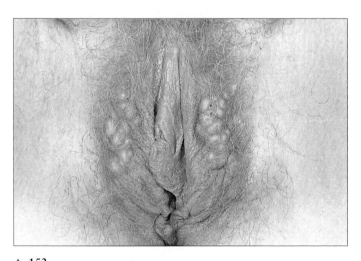

▲ 152
(a) What physical sign is shown?
(b) What treatment is required?

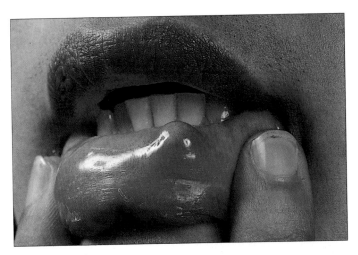

▲ 153
This lesion was of recent appearance. What is the diagnosis?

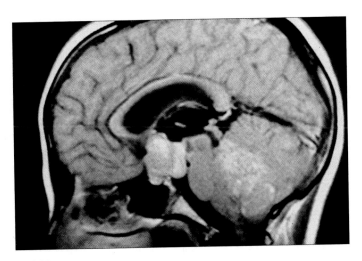

▲ 154
(a) What abnormality is shown on this magnetic resonance imaging (MRI) scan?
(b) List two potential diagnoses.

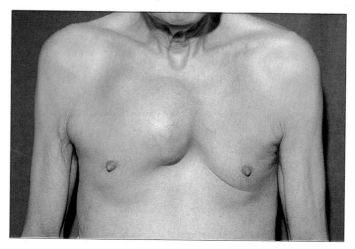

▲ 155
This swelling was pulsatile. What is the likely diagnosis?

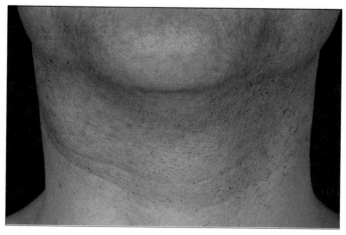

▲ 156
This lump had been present in the neck and had not changed in size over four decades. What is the most likely diagnosis?

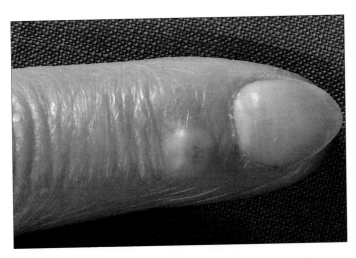

▲ 157
What lesion is shown?

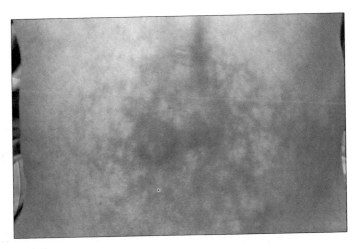

▲ 158
(a) What physical sign is shown on this patient's back?
(b) In what endocrine condition may it occur?

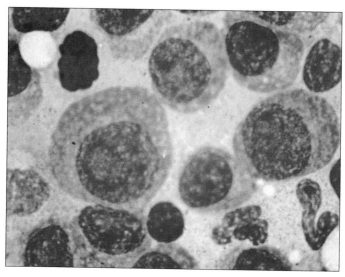

▲ 159
This is a bone marrow smear from a patient with hypercalcaemia.
What is the diagnosis?

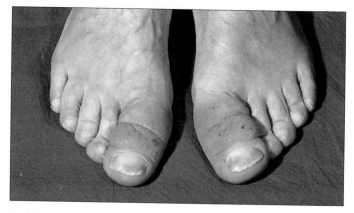

▲ 160
This person's hands had a similar appearance. What is the
diagnosis?

161 ▶
What is the most
likely cause of this
appearance?

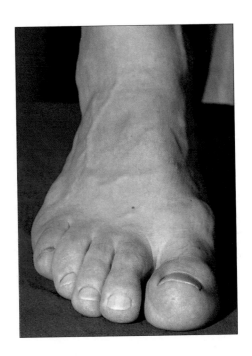

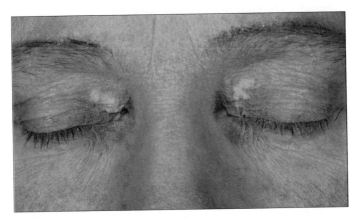

▲ 162
(a) What physical sign is shown?
(b) List two associations.

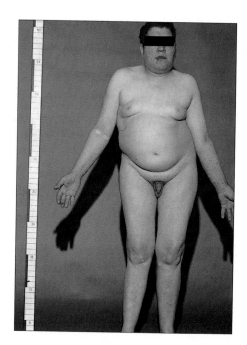

◀ **163**
This man presented with gynaecomastia. He was found to be tall, but otherwise of normal intelligence. What is the most likely diagnosis?

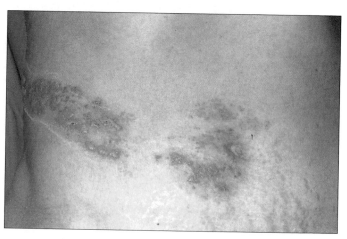

▲ **164**
What is the most likely cause of this lesion?

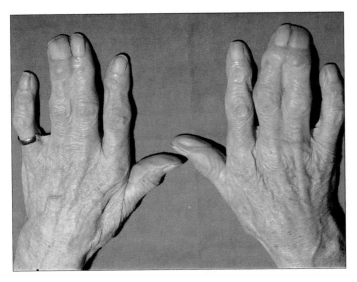

▲ 165
(a) What physical signs are shown?
(b) List two potential causes.

166 ▶
What is the most
likely cause of this
appearance?

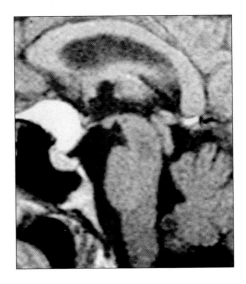

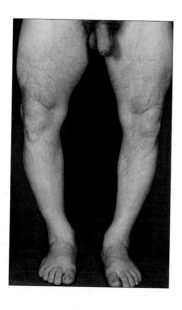

(a) What is the most likely cause
of this appearance?
(b) List two possible underlying
diagnoses.

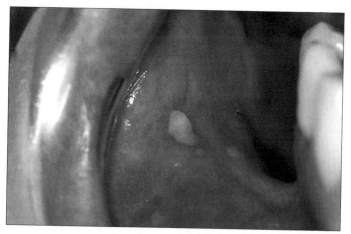

▲ 168
This lesion was found in the mouth of a patient being investigated
for an iritis. The lesion was painful. What is the likely underlying
diagnosis?

169 ▶

These are the genitalia of a 57-year-old man with anosmia.
(a) What physical sign is shown?
(b) What is the likely underlying diagnosis?

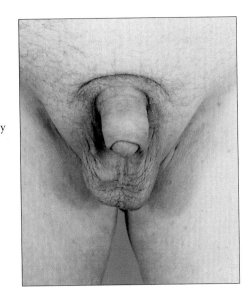

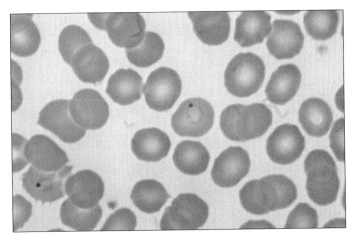

▲ **170**

This is the blood film of a patient returning from vacation in India. She had a febrile illness shortly before presentation.
(a) What is the diagnosis?
(b) What is the treatment?

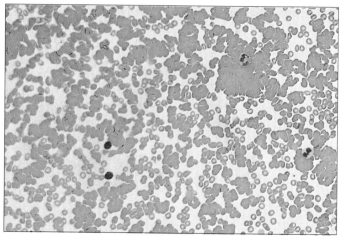

▲ 171
This is the blood film of a patient with a recent atypical chest infection. What diagnosis is suggested?

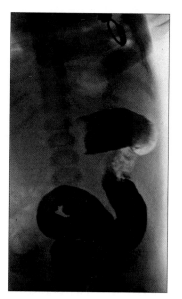

◄ 172
This barium contrast study was performed in a child with abdominal pain and blood in the stool. What abnormality is shown?

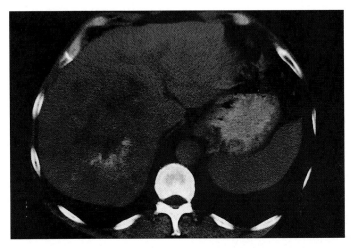

▲ 173
What abnormality is shown on this computerized tomography (CT) scan?

174 ▶
What diagnosis is suggested by this computerized tomography (CT) scan appearance?

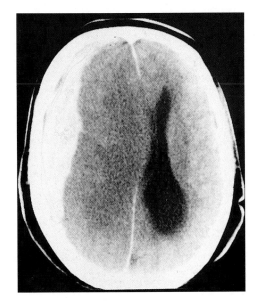

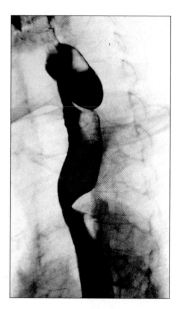

◄ 175
This patient has two causes of dysphagia. What are they?

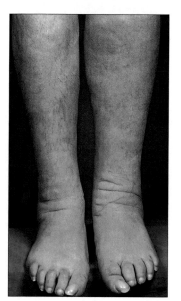

◄ 176
These itchy indurated lesions have been present for a five-year period. The patient had neck surgery some ten years ago. What is the likely diagnosis?

177 ▶

What abnormality is shown on
this contrast-enhanced
computerized tomography (CT)
scan?

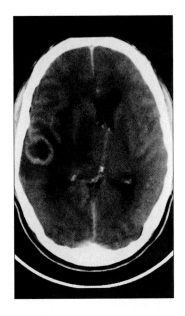

178 ▶

(a) What abnormality is shown?
(b) Suggest two possible causes.

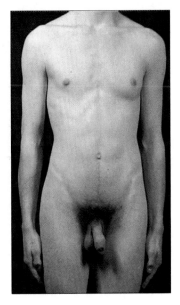

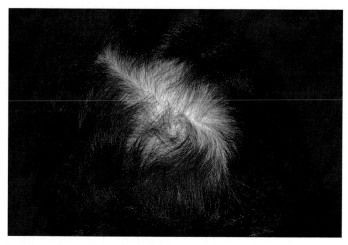

▲ 179

This is the scalp of a patient who complains of weight gain and a general lethargy and lack of vitality. What underlying cause should be sought?

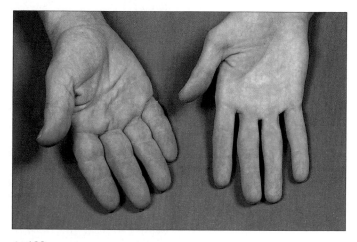

▲ 180

The hand on the right of the picture is a normal hand. What is the diagnosis on the left?

181 ▶

What diagnosis is suggested by
this man's appearance?

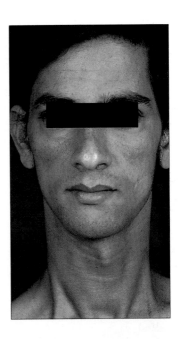

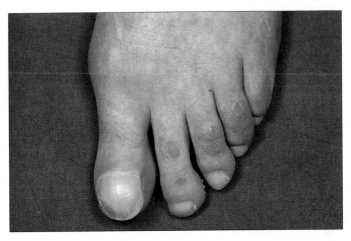

▲ 182

These are the feet of the patient in **181**. What diagnosis is
suggested?

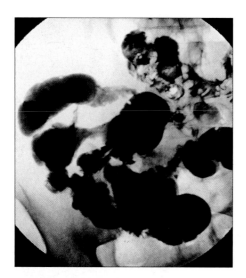

◄ 183
This patient was investigated for weight loss and colicky abdominal pain. What is the likely diagnosis?

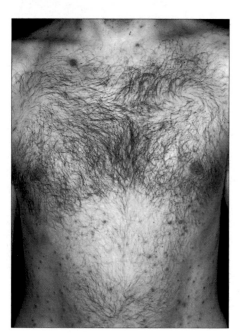

◄ 184
This papulosquamous rash was associated with generalized lymphadenopathy and some ulcerated lesions in the mouth. What diagnosis is suggested?

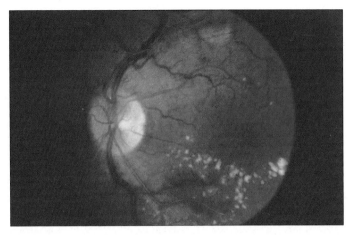

▲ 185
What is the most likely cause of this fundal appearance?

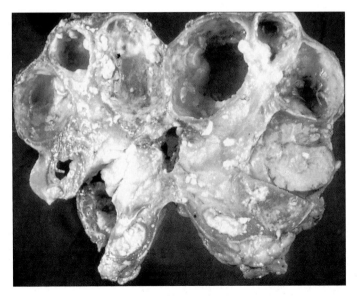

▲ 186
What is the likely cause of the appearance of these kidneys?

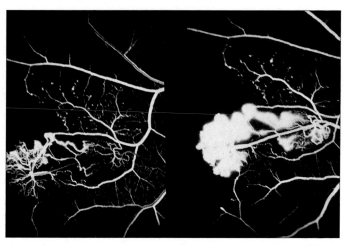

▲ 187
This fluorescence study was performed in a patient with known anaemia. What is the cause of the appearance?

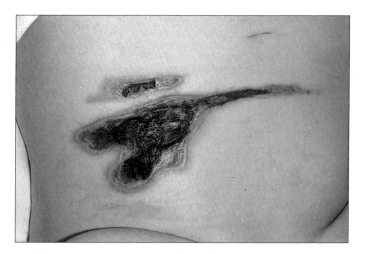

▲ 188
This is the skin of a woman who was found unconscious on the floor. What is the likely cause of this appearance?

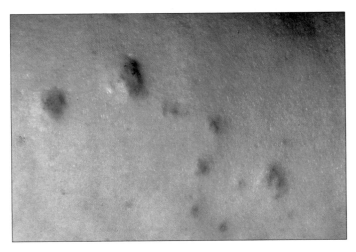

▲ 189
What lesions are these?

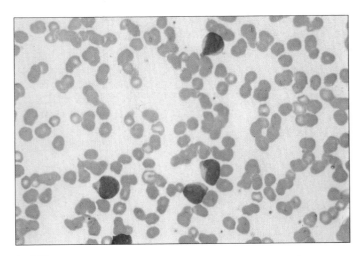

▲ 190
What haematological diagnosis is suggested by this blood film,
taken from an anaemic child with a tendency to bleed?

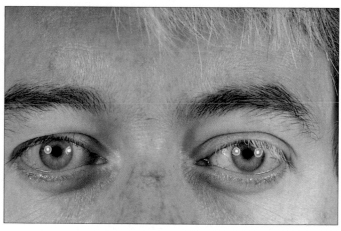

▲ 191
(a) What physical sign is shown?
(b) Cite one associated endocrinopathy.

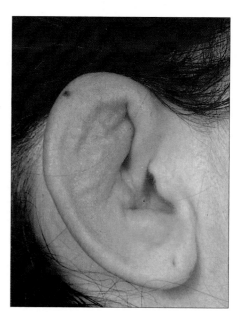

◀ 192
This patient had recurrent episodes of soreness in the ear associated with polyarthritis and microscopic haematuria. What diagnosis is suggested?

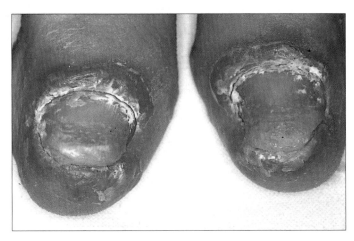

▲ 193
What is the most likely cause of this appearance?

194 ▶
This man, a heavy smoker, complained of considerable breathlessness and a fullness in his face. What is the most likely cause of his appearance?

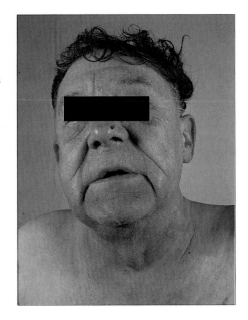

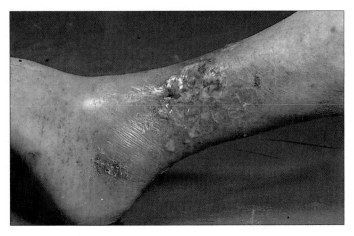

▲ 195
What is the most likely cause of this chronic ulcerative lesion?

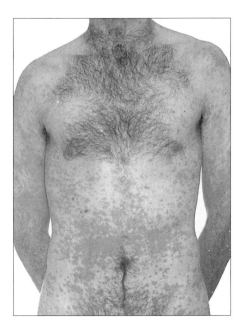

◀ 196
This is the appearance of a man who had recently been put on dapsone for a gastrointestinal condition. What diagnosis is suggested?

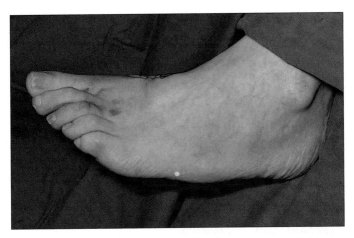

▲ 197
What is the likely cause of this appearance?

198 ▶
This man suffered
from headaches.
What physical signs
should be sought as
a matter of
urgency?

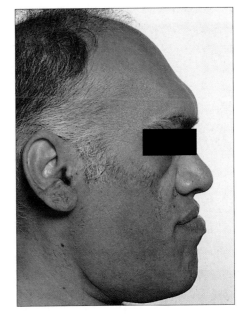

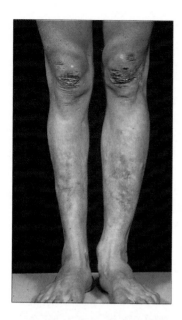

This is the appearance of a patient in whom considerable joint hyperlaxity could be demonstrated. What is the likely underlying diagnosis?

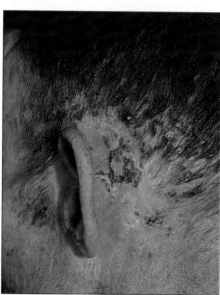

◀ 200
What is the most likely cause of this appearance?

1 (a) Myxoedema.
(b) Serum total thyroxine (T_4), thyroid stimulating hormone (TSH), thyroid antibodies.

2 (a) Arachnodactyly (Marfan's) syndrome.
(b) Dislocation of the lens may case monocular diplopia. Patients with Marfan's syndrome are usually tall and have long limbs compared with other members of the same family. Fingers and hands are slender and have a spider-like appearance. Many patients have severe chest deformities including pectus excavatum, pectus carinatum or asymmetry. Scoliosis is usually accompanied by kyphosis. Dislocation of the lens can occur in both Marfan's syndrome and homocystinuria. Altered collagen in the suspensory ligament accounts for the dislocation.

3 (a) Pseudohypoparathyroidism.
(b) Type 1 pseudohypoparathyroidism is an inherited disorder characterized by target organ-resistance to parathyroid hormone (PTH). Many patients also exhibit partial resistance to other hormones acting by stimulation of adenyl cyclase such as thyroid stimulating hormone (TSH), vasopressin and glucagon. In one variant of the disorder (type 1A) the molecular defect results in reduced cellular concentration of the alpha subunit of the stimulatory protein G ($G_{s\alpha}$), and this partial deficiency is due to lower cellular levels of the mRNA that encode the polypeptide. Pseudohypoparathyroidism type 1B is a similar syndrome in which cellular concentration of $G_{s\alpha}$ is normal. Shortening of the fourth or fifth metacarpals is characteristic of the syndrome.

4 (a) Acromegaly. She shows the typical coarsened features with enlarged nose and pronounced skin markings, and snoring may be caused by macroglossia and increased soft tissue bulk in the pharynx.
(b) Typically there is a failure of an oral glucose tolerance test to suppress circulating growth hormones (50% have a paradoxical rise in growth hormones) and insulin-like growth factor 1 (IGF1) levels are generally elevated, but correlate poorly with the activity of the disease.

5 (a) Pellagra. Patients with pellagra have a brown discoloration of the skin, especially in some exposed areas, as a result of nicotinic acid deficiency. In the areas of increased pigmentation, there is a thin varnish-like scale. These changes are also seen in patients who are vitamin B_6 deficient, have functioning carcinoid tumours (increased consumption of niacin) or take isoniazid.
(b) Pellagra is caused by niacin deficiency. This is a generic term for nicotinic acid (pyridine-3-carboxylic acid) and derivatives exhibiting the nutritional activity of nicotinic acid. The vitamin is absorbed rapidly from the intestine by both active and passive transport mechanisms. Niacin is the essential component of nicotinamide adenine dinucleotide (NAD) and nicotinamide adenine dinucleotide phosphate (NADP), the coenzymes for many oxidation–reduction reactions.

6 (a) Von Recklinghausen's disease. The chest shows the characteristic features of this neurocutaneous disorder with café-au-lait spots.

(b) The disorder may be associated with tumours within the central nervous system including optic glioma, glioblastoma, meningioma and, more rarely, phaeochromocytomas. Other associated aberrations include hamartomas of the iris (Lisch nodules), freckling (particularly within the axillae), macrocephaly unassociated with hydrocephalus and stenosis of the aqueduct of Sylvius leading to obstructed hydrocephalus. Type 1 neurofibromatosis is carried on chromosome 17 and is due to a defect of the encoded protein neurofibromin. Neurofibromatosis type 2 is carried on chromosome 22 and is also a dominant disorder in which neurofibromas involve the acoustic nerves exclusively and usually bilaterally. The acoustic neuromas may produce deafness and other symptoms and signs of a cerebellopontine angle lesion. They may also be associated with meningiomas and astrocytomas.

7 (a) Clitoromegaly.

(b) Deepening of the voice, acne/hirsuties, androgenic alopecia.

8 (a) Acromegaly.

(b) Hypertension, acromegalic cardiomyopathy, and peripheral vascular disease. Hypertension occurs in about one-third of acromegalic patients and is characterized by suppressed renin and aldosterone secretion, associated with an expansion of plasma volume and total body sodium. Almost all hypertensive acromegalics and about one-half of non-hypertensive acromegalics have an increased ventricular mass or left ventricular wall thickness. A very specific cardiomyopathy may occur and acromegalics may develop congestive cardiac failure in the absence of other known underlying heart disease.

9 (a) Pretibial myxoedema. This manifests as a waxy infiltrative collection of plaques, usually in a patient with underlying Graves' disease.

(b) Topical application of potent fluorinated corticosteroids under occlusive dressings may help.

10 (a) Adenoma sebaceum.

(b) Epilepsy. The lesions of adenoma sebaceum are angiofibromas distributed in a butterfly pattern over the cheeks, chin and forehead. The individual adenomas vary in size from 0.1–1 cm and are elevated and pinkish or pinkish-yellow in colour. The cutaneous lesion may provide the earliest clue to the cause of epilepsy. Rhabdomyomas of the heart and tumourous malformations (angioleiomyomas of the kidney, liver, adrenal glands and pancreas) may also occur in this condition.

11 (a) Tetracycline used systemically.

(b) Systemic use of tetracyclines in children up to eight years of age causes discoloration of the teeth, which may be permanent. A further recognized complication of tetracycline usage in paediatric age groups is enamel hypoplasia, as well as a decrease in linear skeletal growth rate.

12 (a) Extracapillary (crescenteric) glomerulonephritis is the most likely diagnosis. Idiopathic or primary rapidly progressive glomerular nephritis is not a homogenous disease. By light microscopy, the characteristic abnormality in the kidney is excessive extracapillary proliferation (i.e. crescents), often associated with segmental or diffuse necrotizing lesions of the glomerular capillaries. Capillary-related antigens are nearly always demonstrable within the crescents by special stains or by immuno-fluorescence.

13 Burkitt's lymphoma. This is thought to be an Epstein–Barr virus (EBV)-related neoplasm. In Burkitt's lymphoma, the typical translocation between chromosomes 8 and 14 places the cellular *myc* gene adjacent to the immuno-globulin heavy chain locus, which is a site of gene activation in the normal lymphocyte. EBV is closely associated with African Burkitt's lymphoma as well as nasopharyngeal carcinoma in Asia. Co-factors in the development of these malignancies might be holoendemic malaria in African Burkitt's lymphoma and a particular configuration of the histocompatibility antigens in the case of nasopharyngeal carcinoma among the Chinese.

14 (a) Lingual thyroid.
(b) A technetium or ^{131}I scan will demonstrate uptake in the area of the posterior tongue. Patients are usually euthyroid and no specific therapy is required. The origin of the thyroid diverticulum is at the foramen caecum, at the junction of the anterior two-thirds and posterior one-third of the tongue. Failed migration of this diverticulum leads to the *in situ* development of the tongue in this area.

15 (a) Old choroiditis.
(b) A probable central scotoma.

16 (a) This is a giant cell epulis.
(b) Surgical removal.

17 (a) Black tongue.
(b) Tetracycline; the use of bismuth salts.

18 This shows buccal pigmentation, which may occur in Addison's disease or haemochromatosis, or be associated with small bowel polyposis.

19 Lichen planus.

20 Gingivitis with mercury blue lines in the gum. The anaemia is likely to be a sideroblastic anaemia.

21 Hutchinson's teeth. These are centrally notched, widely spaced peg-shaped upper central incisors. They are usually associated with mulberry molars that have multiple poorly developed cusps that number more than the usual four. These physical signs are associated with congenital syphilis, other physical signs for which include an abnormal facies, such as frontal bossing, saddle nose, and poorly developed maxillae, with some congenital ectodermal dysplasia.

22 (a) Simian hand crease in Down's syndrome.
(b) A diagnosis is confirmed by karyotyping, which will show the 21 trisomy.

23 (a) Choroidal tear.
(b) High myopia.

24 Coloboma.

25 (a) Scurvy.
(b) Gingival swelling, bleeding, ulceration, and loosening of the teeth may occur in scurvy. Flattened corkscrew hairs with surrounding haemorrhage on the lower extremities are seen in addition to this gingivitis. Vitamin C is a co-factor for lysyl hydroxylase, an enzyme involved in the first translation or modification of procollagen, which is necessary for crosslink formation. In adults, the cardinal features of scurvy include perifollicular hyperkeratotic papules in which hairs become buried. Perifollicular haemorrhages and purpura beginning on the backs of the lower extremities and coalescing to become ecchymoses may occur, as may haemorrhages into joints, splinter haemorrages in the nail base, poor wound healing, and breakdown of recently healed wounds. In infancy and childhood, haemorrhage into the periosteum of long bones causes painful swellings and may result in epiphyseal separation.

26 (a) Multiple haemangiomas of the tongue.
(b) This may be associated with gastrointestinal bleeding and iron deficiency anaemia.

27 (a) Retinitis pigmentosa.
(b) If, as is usual, only the periphery of the retina is involved, there may be loss of navigational vision and the appearance of tunnel vision as the rods degenerate. Recently, it has been demonstrated that mutations of rhodopsin may account for certain forms of retinitis pigmentosa.

28 An acute extradural haematoma from head trauma.

29 Gardner's syndrome. This is a dominantly inherited syndrome comprising multiple adenomatous polyps and adenocarcinomas of the colon as well as of the sphincter of Oddi. Some families also have osteomas, lymphomas, and fibromas.

30 Hypernephroma. This accounts for 85% of all primary renal neoplasms, with a peak incidence at 55–60 years of age and a male:female ratio of 2:1. Environmental risk factors include exposure to cigarette smoke and cadmium. Hereditary forms of renal cell carcinoma, which are often multifocal and bilateral, may occur in a high proportion of patients with von Hippel–Lindau syndrome. The term renal cell carcinoma is now preferred.

31 Turner's syndrome (gonadal dysgenesis). The expected karyotype is XO and patients typically have short stature, rarely reaching more than 150 cm in final height. Rarely, certain mosaics may have spontaneous menses, and then develop the features of primary gonadal failure.

32 (a) Bilateral ptosis.
(b) This may be associated with myasthenia gravis, ocular myopathies, botulinum toxin, bilateral third nerve palsies, or dystrophia myotonica.

33 (a) This shows a simple fissured tongue.
(b) No treatment is required other than reassurance.

34 Tuberculous lymphadenitis.

35 Kallmann's syndrome. A shortened fourth metacarpal is frequently seen in this condition.

36 Hypertensive retinopathy, stage IV. The retina shows evidence of papilloedema and other features of severe hypertensive retinopathy.

37 (a) Macular degeneration.
(b) Diminishing visual acuity. Bruch's membrane is a multilayered structure formed by the choris-capillaris and the pigment epithelium with the retina. With ageing, the latter may accumulate intracellular material leading to age-related macular degeneration. Visual loss is slowly progressive and associated with metamorphopsia. The second type of age-related macular degeneration can occur in the paramacular–foveal area and cause visual loss, resulting from degeneration of Bruch's membrane (with the formation of large or small breaks in its integrity) and subretinal neovascularization. Laser ablation of the neovascular net may delay blindness.

38 (a) Carcinoma of the upper lip.
(b) Tobacco, spicy food.

39 (a) Magnetic resonance imaging (MRI) scan (coronal section) of the hypothalamo-pituitary region.
(b) Microadenoma.
(c) Prolactin estimations should be performed.
(d) Treatment is usually with a dopamine agonist.

40 (a) Herpes zoster of the second division of the trigeminal nerve.
(b) The aetiological agent is a DNA virus (*Varicella zoster*).

41 (a) Central retinal venous occlusion. This may occur as a result of a hyper-viscosity state.
(b) An uncommon complication is the appearance of glaucoma.

42 Choroidal melanoma.

43 (a) Myasthenia gravis.
(b) An edrophonium chloride test may be performed. Ten milligrams of intravenous edrophonium is given and the effect of this short-acting anticholinesterase is assessed. Patients with myasthenia will show an instantaneous improvement in symptomatology, though this is of short duration.

44 (a) This is an exudative detachment of the retina.
(b) Classically, there is an altitudinal field loss.

45 A sixth-nerve palsy on the right. This is a consequence of extension of his tumour towards the apex of the petrous temporal bone (Gradenigo's syndrome).

46 Hypophosphataemic rickets. Rickets and osteomalacia occur in association with a variety of disorders of proximal renal tubular function. These disorders have in common an increased renal clearance of inorganic phosphate with concomitant hypophosphataemia, in association with a normal or near-normal glomerular filtration rate. In hypophosphataemic rickets, lower limb deformities appear and become progressively worse when a child begins to walk and bear weight. The rate of linear growth is at first normal and then slowed. Many of these individuals develop a unique disorder of tendons, ligaments, and joint capsules, characterized by calcification, or more, probably ossification of the insertions of tendons and ligaments and joint capsules (enthesopathy). Hypophosphataemia is due to defective renal conservation of phosphate, which in turn is due to defective phosphate transport across the luminal membrane of proximal renal tubular cells.

47 (a) Pituitary macroadenoma with supersellar extension.
(b) Headaches due to dural stretch and visual field loss are likely.

48 (a) This is advanced diabetic retinopathy.
(b) Simple urine test for glucose or fasting blood sugar is diagnostic.

49 (a) Simple naevus.
(b) No action needs to be taken.

50 (a) The appearance is of a branched retinal venous occlusion.
(b) This may occur spontaneously or in association with hypertension or elevated intraocular pressure. Venous stasis retinopathy can mimic early vein occlusion with venous dilatation, haemorrhages, and cotton wool spots, being due to impaired retinal perfusion produced by severe carotid occlusive disease. Systemic coagulopathy, such as thrombocytopenia, disseminated intravascular coagulopathy, and systemic lupus erythematosus with anti-circulating anti-cardiolipin, may cause retinal haemorrhages.

51 Ocular toxicity due to chloroquine. Irreversible retinal damage may be more likely to occur when the daily dosage of chloroquine equals or exceeds the equivalent of 150 mg base, or 2.4 mg base/kg/day. The drug can also be responsible for ocular toxicity involving the cornea (corneal opacities), keratopathy, and retinopathy.

52 Pendred's syndrome. This is one of a number of defects in which there is defective generation of peroxidase activity on which the oxidation of iodide in the thyroid depends. In Pendred's syndrome, the defective iodination is incomplete and there is an associated nerve deafness. Hypothyroidism, if present, is usually mild. The diagnosis is suspected with an abnormal perchlorate discharge test. Radioactive iodine is given to suspect patients and time allowed for its accumulation by the thyroid gland; its loss from the gland is then observed after oral administration of potassium perchlorate.

53 (a) Herpes simplex infection. Herpes simplex viruses (HSV1 and HSV2; herpes virus hominis) produce a variety of infections involving mucocutaneous surfaces, the central nervous system, and, occasionally, visceral organs. The advent of effective antiviral therapy for HSV infections has made prompt diagnosis of these syndromes of clinical importance. Exposure to the virus at mucosal surfaces or abraded skin permits entry of the virus and initiation of replication in cells of the epidermis and dermis. After infection, nucleocapsid is thought to be transported intra-axonally to the nerve cell bodies and ganglia. During the initial phase of infection viral replication occurs in ganglia and contiguous neural tissue. Virus then spreads to other mucosal skin surfaces through centrifugal migrational infections of virions by peripheral sensory nerves.
(b) Temporal-like encephalitis.

54 (a) Undescended testes.
(b) There is a long-term risk of malignancy in undescended testes, in which there may also be defective spermatogenesis. Some 85% of patients with X-linked Kallmann's syndrome have undescended testes.

55 Reiter's syndrome. This occurs in a sporadic (apparently sexually transmitted) form that usually follows chlamydial infection and in a

postdysenteric form that usually follows infection with the *Yersinia, Campylobacter,* or *Shigella* species. Bilateral conjunctivitis is the commonest eye lesion and is usually mild and of short duration. Anterior uveitis occurs later and is frequently unilateral, though in subsequent attacks alternate eyes may be involved. It tends to recur and become the dominant symptom. The conjunctivitis is not uncommonly painless.

56 Klippel–Feil syndrome. Fusion of two or more spinal vertebrae in this syndrome is associated with a short neck and restricted movement. In addition to the synkinesis, secondary spastic tetraparesis due to subluxation is an occasional complication. The condition may be associated with renal agenesis and is inherited in an autosomal dominant fashion. Winged scapulae may be a feature.

57 (a) Leptospirosis. This should be differentiated from other febrile illnesses, such as enteric fever, rickettsial diseases, glandular fever, brucellosis, and dengue fever, as well as aseptic meningitis. In addition to the jaundice, thrombocytopenia may be present, with increased fibrin degradation products (FDPs) present. Urinalysis may show marked proteinuria and jaundice is of a choloestatic type.
(b) Penicillin, tetracycline, and erythromycin are among the antibiotics capable of killing *Leptospira.* A Jarisch–Herxheimer reaction may occur when penicillin is given early in the course of the disease.

58 Peutz–Jeghers syndrome. This is a syndrome of mucocutaneous pigmentation (circumoral, hands, and feet) and gastrointestinal polyposis, which (like adenomatous polyposis) is inherited as a Mendelian dominant trait. The polyps may occur anywhere in the intestine, but associated malignancy is rare except in the duodenal region in the stomach, where carcinomas may arise. The lip and mouth pigmentation is a useful clinical marker. Prophylactic resection of the small intestine may be advised if polyps over 1 cm in diameter are found on radiographic examination.

59 Lindau's disease. This is associated with haemangioblastomas of the retina (von Hippel's disease), similar lesions in the spinal cord, cysts of the pancreas and kidney, and hypernephromas or tumours of the suprarenal glands. Lindau's disease is familial in approximately 25% of cases.

60 (a) Right pleural effusion and cannonball lesion in the right lung.
(b) Malignancy.

61 (a) Corneal clouding.
(b) This is most commonly associated with the mucopolysaccharidoses, a broad spectrum of disorders due to deficiencies of one of a group enzymes that degrade three classes of mucopolysaccharides: heparan

sulphate, dermatan sulphate, and keratan sulphate. The phenotype includes coarse facies, corneal clouding, hepatosplenomegaly, joint stiffness, hernias, dysostosis multiplex, mucopolysaccharide excretion in the urine, and metachromatic staining in peripheral leucocytes and bone marrow. Corneal clouding is a particularly early feature.

62 (a) Sarcoidosis.
(b) Elevated serum angiotensin-converting enzyme (ACE) level, increased 24-hour urinary calcium, polyclonal gammopathy, hypercalcaemia.

63 (a) Gaucher's disease.
(b) This disease is caused by deficiency of the enzyme glucocerebroside β-glucosidase. There are three clinical types of Gaucher's disease: type 1, chronic non-neuronopathic (adult); type 2, acute neuronopathic (infantile); type 3, subacute neuronopathic (juvenile). All patients have hepatosplenomegaly and large 20–100 μm diameter glucocerebroside-containing reticuloendothelial histiocytes in the bone marrow. The condition is associated with avascular necrosis of the femoral neck.

64 (a) Bilateral retinoblastoma.
(b) Evidence for a recessive mechanism in retinoblastoma was suggested by cytogenetic abnormalities, which showed deletions in the long arm of chromosome 13. This is noted in normal as well as tumour cells of some patients. The gene, RB, encodes a 105 kDa nuclear phosphoprotein, which has protein–protein interaction properties. It seems as though loss of the RB protein results in neoplastic transformation and unregulated cell growth. RB acts as a tumour suppressor gene.

65 Use of a leech to eliminate a haematoma. This method is occasionally used for haematomas of the ear. Medicinal leeches can only be used once, however, because of the risk of transmission of diseases such as Hepatitis B, C, HIV, etc. The animal is placed on the skin and sinks its hooks into the lesion, with the help of a sweet solution applied to the skin. Once the haematoma has been aspirated, irrigating the contact point with hypertonic saline releases the animal from the skin.

66 (a) Carbuncle.
(b) *Staphylococcus aureus* is the likely organism. Staphylococcal infection within the thick fibrous inelastic skin of the back of the neck and upper part of the back leads to formation of a carbuncle. The relative thickness and impermeability of the overlying skin allows lateral extension and loculation, and a large indurated painful lesion with multiple ineffective drainage sites results. Carbuncles produce fever, leucocytosis, extreme pain, and prostration, and bacteraemia is common.

67 Vasculitis. These nailfold infarcts may occur in the context of bacterial endocarditis, dermatomyositis, and a variety of other vasculitides.

68 (a) Gouty tophus.

(b) Hyperuricaemia is the underlying biochemical abnormality. This is the tophaceous form of gout, with the deposition of uric crystals in the ear. Hyperuricaemia can result from increased production of urate or decreased excretion of uric acid, or a combination of the two processes. When hyperuricaemia exists, plasma and extracellular fluids are supersaturated with urate and conditions exist that favour crystal formation and tissue deposition.

69 Aphthous ulceration. Aphthous ulcers resemble cancre sores of the mouth, and in approximately 5–10% of patients they are present during periods of active inflammatory bowel disease and can then resolve during phases of disease inactivity. The commonest cause of aphthous ulceration is simple trauma to the mouth.

70 (a) Clitoromegaly. Prominent labial folds.

(b) Clitoromegaly may be associated with androgen excess in a female, due to either ovarian or adrenal overproduction. It may also occur in severe polycystic ovarian syndrome and following androgen intake by women.

71 Anthrax. This is an acute bacterial infection caused by *Bacillus anthracis*, humans becoming infected when spores are introduced into the body by contact with infected animals or contaminated animal products, insect bites, inhalation, or ingestion. In cutaneous anthrax, a localized skin lesion has a central eschar surrounded by marked non-pitting oedema. Inhalation anthrax typically causes haemorrhagic mediastinitis, a rapidly progressive systemic infection with a high mortality.

72 This is a ranula. Typically, the patient may state that the swelling has appeared before and burst, perhaps several times. The examination of the patient should exclude the possibility of a deep prolongation of the cyst by palpation beneath the mandible. Complete excision or partial excision with marsupialization is appropriate.

73 (a) Ankylosing spondylitis.

(b) Human lymphocyte antigen (HLA) B27 gene product. The spondylo-arthropathies are a group of disorders that show certain clinical similarities. In addition, each of these conditions is associated with the expression of the HLA B27 gene product. The similarity in clinical manifestations and in genetic predisposition suggests that the spondyloarthropathies may have a related pathogenic mechanism. The disorders include ankylosing spondylitis, Reiter's syndrome, reactive arthritis, psoriatic arthritis, and spondylitis. Ankylosing spondylitis is an inflammatory disorder of unknown cause that primarily affects the axial skeleton or the peripheral joints; extraarticular structures may also be involved.

74 Tuberculous lymph node.

75 (a) Left Horner's syndrome.
(b) Typically, this causes ptosis, anhidrosis, miosis, enophthalmos and dilatation of the conjunctival vessels on the same side.

76 Gout. This is caused by the deposition of sodium biurate crystals in the joint.

77 (a) Kleinfelter's syndrome.
(b) The diagnosis is established by performing a karyotype, which will show the typical XXY pattern. Testicular biopsy will reveal an almost Leydig cell-only appearance with dysgenesis and hyalinization of seminiferous tubules.

78 (a) Hirsutism
(b) Probably corticosteroid-induced.

79 Pilonidal sinus.

80 (a) Stevens–Johnson syndrome.
(b) This may be associated with the intake of several drugs, including sulphonamides, barbiturates, chlorpropamide, and the anticonvulsant phenytoin.

81 (a) Cervical lymphadenopathy.
(b) A fine needle aspiration is indicated.

82 (a) Carcinoid flush (syndrome).
(b) Typically, there will be an elevation of the 5-hydroxyindoleactetic acid metabolite in the urine.

83 (a) The appearances are those of papilloedema, showing swelling of the optic disc resulting from elevated intracranial pressure. The condition is typically bilateral, but often asymmetrical, and associated with transient visual loss, optic atrophy, and impaired vision; field loss may ensue if papilloedema becomes chronic.
(b) Papilloedema may occur in the context of increased intracranial pressure caused by mass lesions, inflammatory disease, or idiopathic pseudotumour cerebri.

84 (a) Necrotizing vasculitis (e.g. polyarteritis nodosa).
(b) The diagnosis may be confirmed by muscle biopsy or visceral angiography.

85 (a) Myasthenia gravis.
(b) This may be associated with a thymoma and a computerized tomography (CT) scan is suggested.

86 Occlusion of the superior temporal branch of the retinal artery. This may occur as a result of embolization or spontaneous thrombosis.

87 Cat scratch disease. This should be suspected if the patient has lymphadenopathy, exposure to a cat, and a skin lesion at the site of inoculation. The diagnosis may be confirmed by pathological examination of the involved nodes. Typical pathology includes granulomas, central necrosis of the germinal centres, and infiltration by neutrophils. Cat scratch disease appears to be caused primarily by *Rochalimaea henslae*, a small polymorphic gram-negative bacillus that has been diagnosed in the excised lymph nodes of patients. Tender regional lymphadenopathy will persist for more than three weeks, frequently preceded by a skin lesion after contact with cats. It is associated with their erythema nodosum.

88 (a) Xanthelasma.
(b) This may be associated with familial hypercholesterolaemia as well as primary biliary cirrhosis.

89 Actinomycosis. This is caused by a filamentous gram-positive bacteria, which causes a chronic suppuration, with external sinuses that often discharge tiny columns of organisms, referred to as sulphur granules because of their resemblance to elemental sulphur particles. The indolent course resembles that of fungal infections, tuberculosis, or even malignancy. Most abdominal actinomycotic lesions are preceded by surgery (e.g. laparotomy for acute appendicitis). Infection usually begins in the gastro-intestinal tract and spreads to the peritoneal cavity and abdominal wall or extends paracaecally to the subphrenic spaces or pouch of Douglas.

90 (a) Neck webbing associated with Turner's syndrome.
(b) The diagnosis is confirmed by karyotyping, showing an XO chromosomal configuration. Other features of Turner's syndrome include short stature, primary amenorrhoea, ovarian dysgenesis, low-set posterior hairline, increased carrying angle, coarctation of the aorta, widely spaced nipples, renal anomalies, and skeletal dysplasia.

91 Type II hyperlipidaemia. The hands show tendinous xanthomas, which are typical of this condition.

92 (a) Exophthalmos due to dysthyroid eye disease.
(b) Other ocular features include external ophthalmoplegia, optic neuronitis, retinal oedema, raised ocular pressure, exposure keratitis, and orbital lymphoedema.

93 (a) Male escutcheon.
(b) This is most frequently associated with the polycystic ovarian syndrome, which can cause oligo- or secondary amenorrhoea. It is associated with hirsuties, acne, and greasy skin, and usually secondary infertility.

94 (a) This shows the circinate maculopathy caused by diabetes mellitus.
(b) In view of the critical site of the lesion, fluorescein angiography is recommended. The patient should certainly be referred to an ophthalmologist.

95 (a) Striae.
(b) This may occur in the context of Cushing's syndrome, either iatrogenic or spontaneous. In the spontaneous variety, loss of circadian rhythm and elevated urinary free cortisols would be expected.

96 (a) Plexiform neurofibromatosis.
(b) This may be associated with an acoustic neuroma, which in this case was causing a mass effect in the cerebellopontine angle.

97 Thalassaemia major. The 'hair on end' appearance and general rarefaction of the calvarium is evident. The diploë is thicker because of increased bone marrow activity.

98 Ochronosis. Alkaptonuria is a rare disorder of tyrosine catabolism in which deficiency of homogentisic acid oxidase leads to excretion of large amounts of homogentisic acid in the urine and accumulation of oxidized homogentisic acid in connective tissues (ochronosis). After many years it causes a distinctive form of degenerative arthritis.

99 (a) Testicular feminization.
(b) The complete form of testicular feminization is due to androgen receptor mutations causing androgen resistance.

100 There is an arachnoid cyst in the suprasellar cistern invaginating the floor of the third ventricle.

101 These are the appearances of acute generalized pustulosis.

102 Nelson's syndrome. Her pituitary is producing excessive amounts of adrenocorticotrophic hormone (ACTH). To prevent this condition it is necessary to carry out pituitary irradiation shortly after a bilateral adrenalectomy.

103 Thyroglossal cyst.

104 (a) Blue sclera.
(b) This sign is suggestive of osteogenesis imperfecta, which is an inherited

defect that makes bones brittle because of a generalized decrease in bone mass. The disorder is frequently associated with blue sclera, dental abnormalities (dentinogenesis imperfecta), progressive hearing loss, and a positive family history. Some patients have multiple fractures in infancy and childhood, improve after puberty, and fracture more frequently in later life. The blueness of the sclera is probably caused by thinness of the collagen layers of the sclera, allowing the choroid layers to be seen. It should be noted, however, that blue sclera are an inherited trait in some families without evidence of increased bone fragility.

105 Pericardial effusion.

106 Hypertrophic obstructive cardiomyopathy. Systolic anterior motion of the mitral valve anterior leaflet is demonstrable and the interventricular septum is thicker than would be expected normally.

107 Acute myeloid leukaemia.

108 Leishmaniasis. Leishman–Donovan bodies are demonstrated. Bone marrow aspirate and trephine are positive in over 85% of cases. Pentavalent antimonials are highly effective against *Leishmania* and are relatively non-toxic.

109 (a) Chronic tophaceous gout.
(b) Urate crystals may form in the urinary system and cause an obstructive uropathy.

110 The appearance is that of acute glandular fever. A fine petechial rash can be seen on the soft palate, and there is a necrotic debris on the tonsillar bed.

111 (a) Palmar erythema.
(b) This may be associated with chronic liver disease, thyrotoxicosis, rheumatoid arthritis, pregnancy, and the contraceptive pill.

112 Conn's adenoma. The canary-yellowness of the tumour is typical and, characteristically, hypokalaemia is associated with alkalosis, a fully suppressed plasma renin, and normal or elevated aldosterone.

113 Cilioretinal artery occlusion.

114 Phakoma of the retina.

115 (a) Hypermobility of the joints.
(b) This may occur in the context of either Marfan's syndrome or Ehlers–Danlos syndrome, as well as in osteogenesis imperfecta. All three are disorders of collagen synthesis.

116 (a) Porphyria cutanea tarda (PCT). Cutaneous photosensitivity is the major clinical feature. Hypertrichosis and hyperpigmentation, particularly of the face, and thickening, scarring, and calcification, resembling the cutaneous changes of systemic sclerosis may occur. Hepatic uroporphobilinogen decarboxylase deficiency occurs in all types of PCT.

117 Diabetic dermopathy (shin spots). These are generally located over the anterior tibial surface. The lesions are small rounded plaques with a raised border, which may cross at the edges and ulcerate centrally. Several plaques may be arranged in a linear fashion. Pigmentation is not prominent early, but as the lesion heals a depressed scar occurs, with diffuse brown discoloration.

118 Neuropathic joint. This may occur in diabetes mellitus, syringomyelia, and leprosy.

119 (a) Bitot's spots.
(b) These suggest vitamin A deficiency. Night blindness is the earliest symptom of vitamin A deficiency, followed by degenerative changes in the retina. The bulbar conjunctivae become dry (xerosis) and small grey plaques with foamy surfaces develop. These Bitot's spots are reversible with vitamin A treatment. The more serious effects of deficiency are ulceration and necrosis of the cornea (keratomalacia) leading to perforation, endophthalmos, and blindness.

120 Hypercalcaemia. There is a calcium deposit at the sclerolimbic junction and the patient should be investigated for hypercalcaemia. Causes include sarcoidosis and primary hyperparathyroidism.

121 (a) Dysthyroid eye disease in association with thyrotoxicosis.
(b) There is orbital lymphoedema, and congestive changes are seen in both eyes, particularly on the right, with evidence of chemosis.

122 The patient has unilateral gynaecomastia. This may persist from pubertal gynaecomastia, although it may occur *de novo* in the presence of an increased free oestrogen:testosterone ratio. It is particularly important to rule out a human chorionic gonadotrophin (HCG)-producing tumour, as well as an oestrogen-producing tumour of the testis (Leydig cell tumours) and an oestrogen-secreting adrenal lesion.

123 (a) Striae.
(b) Cushing's syndrome.

124 Primary biliary cirrhosis. This shows granulomatous destruction of bile ducts, which is absolutely typical of primary biliary cirrhosis.

125 Roth's spots. These are oval retinal haemorrhages with a clear pale centre and are seen in less than 5% of patients with subacute bacterial endocarditis. However, they are not specific for this condition, and may occur in connective tissue disease and severe anaemia.

126 Pretibial myxoedema. The dermopathy usually associated with Graves' disease is that of pretibial myxoedema and occurs over the dorsum of the legs or feet. It occurs in patients with past or present Graves' disease and is not a manifestation of hyperthyroidism. About one-half of cases occur during the active stage of thyrotoxicosis. The affected area is usually demarcated from normal skin by being raised, thickened, and having an indurated appearance, and may be pruritic and hyperpigmented. The lesions are usually discrete, assuming a plaque-like or nodular configuration, but in some cases are confluent. Clubbing of the fingers and toes, with characteristic bone changes that differ from those of hypertrophic pulmonary osteoarthropathy, may accompany the dermal changes (thyroid acropachy). Treatment is with betnovate ointment under an occlusive dressing.

127 Chronic lymphocytic leukaemia.

128 (a) Keratic precipitates.
(b) It is important to rule out sarcoidosis, syphilis, and tuberculosis.

129 Fanconi syndrome. Dwarfism and hypophosphataemic rickets may occur. Renal failure is rare and the prognosis is good when the systemic manifestations are treated. Typically, there is a swan-necked deformity and cellular atrophy of the initial portion of the proximal tubule, which is probably the anatomical basis of this tubular disorder. The associated defects in the transport of water, sodium, potassium, acid, and phosphate excretion often require treatment. Metabolic acidosis can be corrected by the administration of alkali, while vitamin D helps promote bone healing. Glycosuria, uricosuria, and tubular proteinuria do not need therapy.

130 (a) Circinate maculopathy. The probable underlying diagnosis is diabetic retinopathy.

131 (a) Ectopia lentis.
(b) This is associated with Marfan's syndrome and homocystinuria. The associated symptom is that of monocular diplopia.

132 (a) Paget's disease; it shows bowing of the tibia and massive uptake in the skull.
(b) Characteristically, it is associated with raised bony alkaline phosphatase. Treatment may consist of calcitonin with or without a bisphosphonate compound.

133 (a) Dermatographism. The underlying diagnosis is one of a physical urticaria. The common physical urticarias include dermatographism, solar urticaria, cold urticaria, and cholinergic urticaria.
(b) Patients with dermatographism exhibit linear wheals following minor pressure or scratching of the skin. It is a common disorder affecting approximately 5% of the population. Solar urticaria characteristically occurs within minutes of sun exposure and is a skin sign of the systemic disease erythropoietic protoporphyria. Treatment of dermatographism is usually with antihistamines.

134 Ruptured rectus abdominus muscle. There is a massive haematoma entrapped within the rectus sheath causing this patient's severe anaemia. She had fallen on her way to the toilet.

135 (a) Perl's stain for iron has been performed.
(b) The features are those of haemochromatosis with cirrhosis.

136 Spherocytosis. The major clinical features of hereditary spherocytosis are anaemia, splenomegaly, and jaundice. The latter is due to an increased concentration of unconjugated (indirect reacting) bilirubin in the plasma. Jaundice may be intermittent and tends to be less pronounced in early childhood. Compensatory normoblastic hyperplasia of the bone marrow occurs, with extension of the bone marrow into the midshafts of long bones, and occasionally with extramedullary haemopoiesis, at times leading to the formation of paravertebral masses, which are clearly visible on the chest radiograph. A prominent increase in the osmotic fragility of red cells following sterile incubation of whole blood for 24 hours at 37°C is also characteristic of this condition.

137 Acute gout causing an olecranon bursitis. The thiazide diuretic led to acute hyperuricaemia in this susceptible individual and precipitated acute gout. The differential diagnosis here includes acute septic monoarthritis and other crystal arthropathies.

138 Henoch–Schönlein (anaphylactoid) purpura.

139 Sea fan proliferation demonstrated here occurs in sickle cell diseases (SS, SC, SL).

140 Multiple bone metastases. If radionuclide uptake is increased throughout the entire skeleton, a potential differential diagnosis is osteomalacia with multiple pseudofractures. This is less likely in this instance, however.

141 (a) Pinguecula.
(b) This is associated with Gaucher's disease.

142 (a) Severe acanthosis nigrans. This is a mossy hyperpigmented thickened skin lesion, which is most typically present in skin fold areas in the axillae or groin.
(b) It can occur in patients with obesity, portoscovera syndrome, and insulin resistance. Some patients with acanthosis nigrans show normal to mild glucose intolerance with a compensatory increase in insulin secretion, which is only detected when insulin levels are measured.

143 (a) This is a non-caseating granuloma.
(b) The underlying diagnosis is probably sarcoidosis.

144 This shows a resected adrenal tumour and could be a phaeochromocytoma or, more likely, a Conn's adenoma.

145 Aphthous ulceration in association with ulcerative colitis.

146 Diabetes mellitus with a perforating neuropathic ulcer.

147 Myxoedema. There are a large variety of neurological associations with myxoedema, including drop attacks and ataxia. This patient was found to have undetectable thyroxine (T_4) and greatly elevated thyroid stimulating hormone (TSH).

148 (a) A left seventh nerve lower motor neurone palsy.
(b) Possible causes include Ramsay Hunt syndrome, mononeuritis multiplex, and sarcoidosis.

149 Congenital syphilis or Wegener's granulomatosis. In this particular case the patient had congenital syphilis. Other features that should be sought include Hutchinson's teeth (central notching of the central upper incisors due to defective development of the middle column of cells of the permanent incisors *in utero*) and Moon's molars (the first molar tooth shows poorly developed cusps). The face is characteristically flat due to underdevelopment of the maxillae. In addition, there may be frontal bossing (Parrot's nodes), a saddle nose, as in this instance, and rhagades (linear scars radiating from the angle of the mouth and side of the nose).

150 (a) Ulnar nerve palsy.
(b) Possible causes include injury at the elbow and mononeuritis.

151 (a) This a cavernous haemangioma. It can be associated with platelet consumption (Kasabach–Merritt syndrome), and other musculoskeletal defects.
(b) The lesions tend to resorb spontaneously within 4–5 years

152 (a) Multiple sebaceous cysts of the vulva.
(b) No specific treatment is required unless they become infected. They may be curetted.

153 Mucous cyst of the lips. It is entirely benign.

154 (a) Suprasellar mass invading the hypothalamus.
(b) This turned out to be a tuberculoma of the hypothalamus, but it could also be a secondary deposit in this area.

155 Expanding ascending aortic aneurysm. This is most likely related to syphilitic aortitis.

156 Bronchial cyst.

157 Simple synovial cyst.

158 (a) Erythema ab igne.
(b) This is not infrequently seen in patients with myxoedema.

159 Multiple myeloma. The shows dysmature plasma cells.

160 Thyroid acropachy

161 Acromegaly. There is acral enlargement and considerable increase in the soft tissue content of the foot.

162 (a) Xanthelasmata.
(b) This may occur either in familial dislipidaemic syndromes or alternatively in primary biliary cirrhosis.

163 Kleinfelter's syndrome (XXY) (seminiferous tubule dysgenesis). Characteristic features include tall stature, normal underdeveloped penis, small pea-sized testes, and gynaecomastia.

164 Shingles. This is a recurrence of a herpes zoster infection.

165 (a) Syndactyly, together with osteoarthritis and small muscle wasting.
(b) Syndactyly can occur in association with etretinate administration during pregnancy and ketoconazole administration during pregnancy.

166 Aneurysm of the internal carotid artery at the siphon.

167 (a) Old rickets.
(b) This may be either nutritional or due to old renal disease.

168 Behçet's disease. Recurrent aphthous ulcerations are a *sine qua non* for the diagnosis. The ulcers are usually painful, 2–10 mm in diameter, and shallow or deep with a central yellowish necrotic base. They persist 1–2 weeks and then subside without leaving scars. Genital ulcers resemble the oral ones. Eye involvement is the most dreaded complication as it occasionally progresses rapidly to blindness. Eye disease is usually present at the outset, but may also develop in the first few years. In addition to iritis, posterior uveitis, retinal vein occlusions, and optic neuritis can be seen in some cases. Hypopyon uveitis, which is considered the hallmark of Behçet's syndrome, is in fact rare.

169 (a) Infantile genitalia with poorly developed scrotum and absence of secondary sexual characteristics.
(b) The diagnosis is olfacto genital dysplasia (Kallmann's syndrome).

170 (a) *Plasmodium vivax* infection. This causes a tertian fever. *P. vivax* infection, like *P. ovale* infection, has a phase of illness during which intrahepatic forms are present. These may remain dormant for months before reproduction begins. These hypnozoites cause relapses that characterize infection with these two species.
(b) Chloroquine and primaquine in combination will eliminate the organism.

171 Cold agglutinin formation, probably secondary to *Mycoplasma pneumoniae* infection. Transient cold agglutinins occur commonly in two infections: *M. pneumoniae* infection and infectious mononucleosis. In both the titre of antibody is usually too low to cause clinical symptoms, but its presence is of diagnostic value. Other settings in which cold agglutinins occur include monoclonal antibodies as the product of lymphocytic neoplasia and polyclonal antibodies in response to infection. In many elderly patients, the neoplasm is benign monoclonal gammopathy and, although chronic, it does not progress and the protein product remains its only manifestation.

172 Intussusception of the large bowel. This may occasionally occur in the context of Henoch–Schönlein purpura in children.

173 This is a calcified metastasis, in this case the primary being in the colon.

174 Subdural haematoma with midline shift and hydrocephalus in the opposite lateral ventricle.

175 The barium swallow shows both a pharyngeal pouch and an external compression of the upper portion of the oesophagus, this time caused by an aberrant right subclavian artery. This causes the symptom of dysphagia lusoria.

176 Pretibial myxoedema.

177 Cerebral abscess with considerable oedema of the ipsilateral hemisphere. Cerebral abscess is not an infrequent complication of cyanotic heart disease with a right to left shunt.

178 (a) Unilateral left gynaecomastia.
(b) This could be drug induced or result from an oestrogen-secreting tumour of either the testis (Leydig cell tumour) or adrenal.

179 Biochemical evidence of myxoedema – raised thyroid stimulating hormone (TSH) and low free thyroxine (T_4). The physical sign shown here is diffuse alopecia, which is not infrequent in severe primary hypothyroidism.

180 Acromegaly. It is important to look for evidence of scars that might be caused by decompression of the carpal tunnel.

181 Graves' disease (thyrotoxicosis). Features include considerable myopathy, staring eyes, and a goitre.

182 Thyroid acropachy, with a clubbed appearance of the toes.

183 Crohn's disease. Multiple strictures are seen in this barium follow-through.

184 Secondary syphilis. The manifestations of secondary syphilis include localized or diffuse symmetrical mucocutaneous lesions and generalized non-tender lymphadenopathy. The healing primary chancre is still present in 50% of cases and the skin rash consists of macular, papular, papulosquamous, and occasionally pustular syphilides, often with one or more forms present simultaneously. Non-patchy hair loss can also occur in secondary syphilis and progressive endarteritis obliterans and ischaemia result in superficial scaling of papules and may eventually lead to central necrosis.

185 Severe hypertension. There are soft exudates, retinal oedema, and multiple haemorrhages. This is a negroid fundus.

186 Gross tuberculous changes with caseating lesions and multiple areas of calcification.

187 This is the sea fan appearance classically seen in sickle cell disease.

188 This appearance represents areas of pressure necrosis. The patient had fallen on her hand and remained unconscious for a number of days.

189 (a) Blue rubber bleb naevus syndrome. This is also known as Maffucci's syndrome and patients with this condition may also have haemangiomas of the gastrointestinal tract, which may bleed, whereas patients with

Maffucci's syndrome have associated dyschondroplasia and osteochondromas.

190 Acute myeloblastic leukaemia.

191 (a) Leucotrichia.
(b) This may be associated with Graves' disease and other organ-specific autoimmune diseases.

192 Relapsing polychondritis. This is an episodic and often progressive inflammatory disorder affecting predominantly the cartilage of the ears, nose, and tracheobronchial tree, as well as the eyes and the ears. Other manifestations include polyarthritis, vasculitis, cardiac abnormalities, skin lesions, and glomerulonephritis. It is an uncommon disorder found in all races, but 30% of patients with relapsing polychondritis have another rheumatological disorder, the most frequent being systemic vasculitis, lupus, or Sjögren's syndrome.

193 Psoriasis affecting the nails. The appearance can be quite similar to that found in onychomycosis, but thimble pitting will be present and other lesions will be present on the body.

194 Superior vena cava obstruction, in this case caused by a tumour of the bronchus. These patients require dexamethasone therapy and a rapid course of irradiation.

195 Chronic varicose ulcer.

196 Toxic erythema. Dapsone may be associated with agranulocytosis, aplastic anaemia, and some serious cutaneous reactions, such as exfoliative dermatitis, toxic erythema, erythema multiforme, toxic epidermal necrolysis, morbilliform and scarlatiniform reactions, and erythema nodosum. The drug should be withdrawn immediately.

197 Lymphangiography. This is undertaken to visualize the lymphatic system in the leg and within the abdomen. Evans blue has been introduced subcutaneously to trace the origin of lymphatic channels.

198 Evidence of visual field defect (tunnel vision). This man clearly has acromegaly.

199 Ehlers–Danlos syndrome. The physical sign shown here is that of cigarette paper skin, which is typical of the Ehlers–Danlos syndrome.

200 Herpes zoster infection. This may cause a seventh nerve palsy, the so-called Ramsay Hunt syndrome.

INDEX

Numbers refer to Question and Answer numbers.